The Young Living Lifestyle. Author: Jordan E. Schrandt.
Front and back cover designed by: Nathan Colba

© 2015 Living It Out, LLC
Published by Living It Out, LLC
Springfield, MO
ISBN # 978-1-5136-055-7

Other Works by this Author: The Young Living Welcome Book

For additional copies of this book visit www.wearelivingitout.com

The Young Living Lifestyle

Our Journey to Wellness

Jordan E. Schrandt

Published by Living It Out, LLC
Springfield, MO
Printed in the USA

Contents

Preface:

This book is about YOU. It's about wherever you are in your life today, right now. Look around you... what do you see? This is your life, your health, your body, your family, your future. YOU.

In the following pages I'll take you through our family's journey to abundant wellness in hopes that it will inspire you to take a closer look at your lifestyle, the products in your home, and the choices you make every day.

Ready to jump in?

#LetsDoThis

Chapter 1

My Journey to a More Natural Lifestyle

When I was little, I remember walking through a field or a forest and being surrounded by nature. I remember my dad teaching me what a scissor-tail swallow looked like on a fence post out in the country. I loved plants, animals and the whole outdoors. I think people are naturally drawn to nature—maybe you LOVE city life, but there's still something about a green plant in a city apartment, the smell of fresh air after being inside all day, driving through a country setting and seeing the sun set over a field or watching a sunrise on the beach. Something about nature just moves us. I really believe this innate desire to have nature around us is because we are "all natural" ourselves... we are drawn to what "works" with our bodies.

I've never met someone who says, "oh my goodness, I just LOVE the smell of latex gloves" or "I would rather be sitting in my office with fluorescent lights *any day* over sitting in the sunshine in a park"... we just *don't* feel the same way about man-made stuff. It doesn't resonate with us nearly as much as the things in nature.

I'm going to give you a little background info on me. I promise it's relevant to how I reached the place I'm in now. I hope that this will meet you where *YOU* are… in *YOUR* home and with *YOUR* lifestyle! Perspective helps take you there. #HangWithMe

I grew up in an agricultural family. My dad was an agriculture education teacher at our high school and we owned a beef cattle farm. I showed pigs at the Missouri State Fair when I was a child, raised flowers for the farmers market in middle school, and worked on a hay hauling crew, built cattle fencing across the farm and "worked cows" all through high school.

Dad encouraged us to be really involved in the FFA. (FFA, or Future Farmers of America, is a leadership development organization for high school students who take agriculture education courses). So I was on competitive teams where we studied and competed in our knowledge in forestry, soil science, agronomy (field crops), grasslands, nursery/landscaping and other subjects.

My sophomore year, I gave an agricultural speech at the Missouri FFA State Convention in favor of genetic modification… and somehow, it was convincing enough to win. (Oh my word…) One of the questions I was asked at the end was, "There is an organic food movement really picking up speed… how does that sector of society deal with the increase of genetically modified foods?" … believe it or not, I answered, "I think we should all be united on this front and everyone should convert to all GMO food so that, together, we can support American agriculture in the best way possible." … ummm, wow.

I was all about American agriculture. (Please don't hear me say that I don't LOVE the FFA, because I totally do… it's an AMAZING leadership organization for youth. But I had only one way of thinking and can totally relate to those folks who are literally on that side of the fence).

In college, I got a Bachelor's of Science degree in Agriculture Communications from Missouri State. I loved my classes in animal and plant science. During that time, I was a state officer for the Missouri FFA Association and traveled around Missouri speaking to high school students about American agriculture. I traveled to Taiwan to study the agriculture industry there, as well. Simultaneously, I was writing for a couple different agriculture publications about farmers and producers around Missouri. I would go to the farm, meet the farmer, and interview him about what he was producing and how.

I also was a student ambassador for the Missouri Farm Bureau Association and learned about the legislative side of agriculture policy. My last year at Missouri State I did a second Ag industry tour in Kansas City (the first was my sophomore year of high school in St. Louis). On both of these tours, we traveled to places like production facilities for all sorts of bread and dessert products, grain bins, locks & dams to see how barges transport food across the country, dairy organizations, soybean organizations, corn producer organizations, marketing firms for agriculture companies… you name it, we saw it… including the company who produced the first genetically modified organisms. (You've heard of them, to be sure.) Yes, we saw the inner workings there as well. I believed this all to be steps in the beautiful process of food production and a part of how American agriculture—surrounded by birds, bees, flowers and trees—was the backbone of America. In a sense, that's true, and we'll get to that in a minute. All in all, I loved then, and still do now, all things related to plants, agriculture and nature... It's just a part of me.

With this love of God's creation in mind, I dreamed of being a wife and mom and how I could incorporate these lifestyles and interests together. I wanted to grow my own herbs and garden, raise chickens, and teach my children to love nature, plants and animals as much as I did. I envisioned this rustic yet cultured farm life that would incorporate all my hearts desires into making me a picture-perfect "June Cleaver-meets-Laura Ingalls Wilder-with a little bit of-Annie Oakley-thrown-in" type of wife and mother.

I'd have at least ten perfectly healthy and happy children who would all pick wildflowers together with me and my mountain-man husband. And of course, we'd all arrive at church on time every Sunday morning, with big bows, neatly pressed collars and cowboy boots. Oh yeah, I had my passions, my pursuits and my plans all figured out.

Oh how funny God is… he has *His* awesome ways, and they're always better than our own.

The Big Life Changes...

After college I moved to New York for a year to be a nanny. I wanted to have some life experience outside of rural Missouri. (Though I missed the sight of hay bales, tractors and fields more than ever.) I lived with two different Italian families over the course of that year and WOW... Italians are SO fun and *so not* like a typical southwest Missouri household! It was there that I realized there was an ENTIRE grocery store dedicated to "organic food" called Whole Foods.

Upon first hearing the name, I imagined whole food maybe meant they sold food in whole form (like a bag of wheat kernels instead of ground up wheat?) Yep, I relate to those who've NEVER bought a single thing "organic".

One day while I was kayaking on the Long Island Sound (the gorgeous water north of Long Island and south of Connecticut) I saw a huge school of ENORMOUS fish swimming under me on all sides. I wrote about it in my journal a few days later. It was May 27, 2009. A few states away on that same day, something happened that changed my life forever and here's how that part of the story began:

In 1996 a sweet couple named Doug and Kim got married in Michigan after meeting in college. They both worked a few years and then had their first baby, a sweet little girl, Brianna. Two years later, they had their first son, Luke. Then another two years—and another daughter, Kayla. The fourth baby would have been right on time two years after that, but was lost to a miscarriage. Soon after, Kim was pregnant again and their fourth child, another girl, was born. They named her Emma.

This was the perfect family: good marriage, great kids. The family was beautiful, healthy, homeschooled, and happy. They had play dates, rode bikes to the park, visited Disney World, and she cooked at home almost every night, the normal American diet. Everything seemed perfect.

Then something happened...

A lump and a diagnosis that changed the normalcy of life and was soon followed by an accidental pregnancy. (Which often accelerates breast cancer). Little Nathan was born at home in February. Three girls. Two boys. Believing for a miracle.

But Kim wasn't feeling well. Spring came, and soon she became more ill—to the point that she couldn't walk. The pain was so severe but she never complained. She stayed at home with her children around her. She read them books and had them sit on her lap.

Finally, Doug insisted they go to the hospital. He supported her as she walked out of the threshold of the home they'd made together and drove away. The doctors said it was only a matter of time so Doug decided to bring the children.

Brianna had just turned nine and was Kim's cooking buddy in the kitchen. "Luke'er" as his mommy called him, had just turned seven. Kayla was in kindergarten… just barely five. Emma was the little cutie pie… at two and a half. Nathan didn't go to the hospital. He was only three and a half months old. Doug dimmed the lights in the hospital room so the children couldn't see her yellowing skin. They all hugged and kissed her and told her they loved her.

Later that day, Doug drove back to the hospital alone. He stayed up with Kim all night and the next morning, holding the hand of her sweetheart, and her dad by her side, she took her final breath and entered the gates of heaven.

Doug immediately lifted his hands in the air and said "Thank you GOD for the time you gave us" and then he wept. He was numb. He drove home, gathered the four older children in the back bedroom and told them that Mommy went home to be with Jesus. The three oldest began to cry and Emma, asked "Why is everybody crying?" She cried herself to sleep on Doug's chest for months, asking for Mommy to come home.

Over the next few months, people came out of the woodwork to support this sweet little family of a widower and his five small children. People brought meals, did in home haircuts, and engaged in play dates. The kids' grandparents were a huge support as well. The outpouring of love made life bearable, but the sting of death is all too real in this life… even though Kim is in her eternal home.

A Second Love and a Season of Change

Summer passed, Doug was busy traveling and keeping the kids occupied with family visits. That same summer, I moved home from New York to Missouri, with the whole world at my doorstep! I sensed limitless opportunities as I turned 23 that fall.

Fast forward a few months to January 2010. I was sitting in the computer lab of Missouri State University working on my Masters in Teaching. I happened to browse onto an old Christian Networking site I was a part of while I lived in New York. Doug was on there, too. He introduced himself and told me within the first two minutes we were talking that he was widowed with five children. I was so intrigued to learn about this man who'd gone through such trial and still held fast to his faith and his desire for wholeness for himself and his children.

We exchanged emails and spent the next several months courting and traveling between Missouri and Michigan to spend time together—all seven of us. I remember one night before I left to go back home, Kayla was crying and said, "Why can't you and daddy just go on more dates so you can hurry up and get married?" to which Emma, who was three, cried out, "No, Miss Jordan can't marry daddy because he's married to my mommy!" Oh my goodness, it broke my heart for her, for me, for Doug, for Kim.

Doug and I were engaged in May; the children were a part of the proposal. They desperately wanted normalcy again even though they didn't completely understand the changes that were taking place in their life. I moved to Michigan that summer to live with Doug's family friends so I could get to know the children better.

We spent our engagement (from May until September) traveling to meet family and friends… and not being "married" even though we had the stressors of people who'd been married for 10 years! It was quite a challenge… many days I wanted to give up and throw in the towel.

I came to the house in the mornings with messes everywhere (already?!?), kids everywhere, needs everywhere, and Kim's "handprints" all over everything. Meanwhile I was planning my wedding and trying to have a somewhat normal engagement. I think we got a total of three kid-free dates during those four months. Even still, I was falling in love with the children and I knew that this was right.

One day I remember telling Brianna (who had just turned 10) that I was ordering wedding napkins for mine and daddy's wedding. I asked her if she wanted to help. She said "Yes, but I have an even better idea!" She ran out of the room and was back a few minutes later with a plastic bag. She said, "Could you just use this?!" … so excited to offer a helpful solution. I opened the bag and saw "Doug & Kim. Two Hearts Become One. August 3, 1996". A bag full of wedding napkins. I thought I was going to throw up. My stomach turned in knots. I tried to smile at Brianna but instead ran to the bathroom and wept.

This was what God had called me to. Life is NOT all about me. It's about other people. I knew in my heart that this was my family… regardless of the challenges.

After we were married in September, life was full of Legos on the floor, dress up, children's books and feeding a small army as I was learning to cook. It was borderline survival mode! We ate whatever was quickest and easiest.

During this time, I began having miscarriages. I spent the next 15 months in and out of my OBGYN's office and seeing a specialist for fertility treatments. I had a surgery for endometriosis, polycystic ovarian syndrome, scar tissue and a D&C after one of the miscarriages.

The emotional mountain of going from single, no children to marrying a widower, having five children on my wedding day and then not being able to stay pregnant was at times almost more than I could bear. Being a second wife is hard. Being a second mom is hard. Knowing Kim got pregnant like clockwork made me resentful. I had nightmares that she came to my house, and Doug told me to leave and that he wanted her to be his wife and the mom of his kids instead of me. It was a real, daily struggle in my mind.

Here's where emotional things play into physical ones: Let me tell ya, folks… if you're emotionally out of whack, your body and health *will* follow. And vice versa. I had some enormous bitterness, resentment and jealousy I was dealing with… and I didn't want to let that go. I had a right to feel that way, right? So I justified my negative feelings.

It wasn't until December 2011, 15 months after we were married, that I made the choice of forgiveness. I called Kim's parents and asked if we could get together at Christmas. I had to let go of the pain of being "second" and believing I was less. What lies we can convince ourselves of! I am honored God called me to this… how awesome to be refined by fire! I look back with thankfulness for the experiences we had in those early years.

Lessons from a First Pregnancy

In January 2012, I was pregnant. I supplemented with progesterone, but I maintained the pregnancy and had a lot of peace in my heart, too.

During my pregnancy, I became increasingly aware of the food I was eating, the chemicals I was cleaning with, and the perfumes, lotions and face care products I put on my skin. I just sensed that those things weren't good for the baby and I read that many of those items cross the placental barrier and the baby can absorb them. I, like most moms, inherently knew to avoid as much of that as possible while pregnant. I remember distinctively the smell of my laundry detergent being absolutely repulsive to me. I could hardly do laundry for the overwhelming scent.

It was the first time that I had ever really considered those things to be "not good for me" … and I wanted to do all that I could to protect the baby growing in my womb! I stopped using perfume and lotions and held my nose anytime I sprayed cleaner.

It was then that I felt a true conviction: I spent so much time and energy avoiding toxic products for my unborn baby and yet was feeding and exposing my other five children to those same things every single day without a second thought—and they were predisposed to cancer at a young age even more than your average children!

I felt what a mother feels—that "mama bear" feeling—that I wanted to protect my children, all six of them, from the damage of toxins. I had no idea what that meant or looked like, but I felt that feeling in my heart and I wanted to try to figure it out. Little did I know that the revelation of true health— beyond the farm life I'd imagined for my future—was right around the corner.

My first born, sixth child was born in October of that year… and around the same time we embarked on a journey that would change our lives forever.

Why History Matters

I met my friend Crystal at a new church we tried that fall. She mentioned that I should try out essential oils to support my new adventures in healthy living… maybe make my own bath salts and use some oils to promote a good night's sleep.

I thought she was a weird hippy. (As I had no concept of what she was talking about!)

Regardless, I tried my first essential oil in September, just weeks before my baby was born. It was an oil blend called Valor. I remember rolling it on thinking, "This doesn't smell like *anything* I've ever smelled before." It was so… raw. I loved it!

That was the first of many oils I bought, used and fell in love with. I was so impressed with them! I ordered a ton of reference materials and books, scoured online resources, and read everything I could get my hands on to learn more about this stuff!

What I learned was absolutely fascinating to me!

Breaking into a whole new world of "natural wellness" coupled with what I knew of the development of the agriculture industry totally changed the way I look at human history, and why *this* history matters!

The first documented reference of essential oils is in Genesis of the Christian Bible.

There are references to oils used in ancient Egypt, Rome and in Eastern cultures of the world. They were used for religious ceremonies, cleansing rituals and supporting remedies for the body.

In the past few centuries, however, essential oil production has become a lost art. Our world has seen tremendous and incredible advancements. In America alone, we've experienced a lot of positive change—the end to slavery, the invention of the automobile, sending a man to the moon and the creation of the World Wide Web.

Arguably, however, we've seen a lot of negative change as well. The turn of the century brought Americans off of farms where they lived and worked simply. To most people at that time, a small, diverse farm was the norm.

For most eras in human history, local communities were self-sustainable. You had a butcher, a baker and a candlestick maker. Food, home goods, and other items were freshly made and locally sourced. If they weren't locally produced, then they were a substance that could naturally maintain its integrity over long distances and periods of time, like essential oils, honey and spices.

But during the industrial revolution in America, these small town farmers and craftsmen flooded bigger cities to work in factories, attend universities, or otherwise pursue the "American Dream".

Mass production became commonplace and replaced small shops and mills where products were meticulously hand crafted. The expansion of the railway, highway and waterway systems paved the way for merchandise (both food and home) to be transported from sea to shining sea… and beyond.

New stores were popping up across the country. Soon, there was a network and infrastructure of production, processing, distribution and marketing of food and fiber products in place.

It was the dawn of a new era of opportunity. And thus, products changed to meet the growing demand. In order for food, home and farm merchandise to maintain its freshness and potency for its trek from farm to table, field to closet, or production plant to the home, many manufacturers began adding stabilizers, artificial flavorings, dyes, synthetic fragrances, filler ingredients, preservatives, and other substances to their products. Though the intention was not to alter the quality of the food, home and farm goods—that was the inevitable result.

Farmers had to add pesticides and herbicides to keep their thousand acre fields from being destroyed by bugs or taken over by weeds. (This wasn't as much of an issue when people had smaller, more manageable, diversified farms where they could tend to them properly).

Today we live in a chemical-laden culture… and these chemicals wreak havoc on our "organic" bodies.

We are not a nation that is getting healthier. The opposite is true, and we are a nation that is now sicker than ever before. Ailments, sicknesses and diseases of all kinds are on the rise.

Here are some interesting facts: Benjamin Franklin and Dr. Thomas Bond founded the first hospital in America, called Pennsylvania Hospital, in May 1751. It was free to those who needed it and was never over-run.

According to the 2014 American Hospital Association Annual Survey, just over two and a half centuries later, there are 6,300 hospitals in America with annual costs of over 859 *billion* dollars[1] and it would seem that these facilities are nearly full—all the time.

Ok, whoa. These are just a few basic facts that tell us... *something has significantly changed in our world.*

Let me stop right here to point out that I am NOT against all things "medical". I don't think hospitals are inherently evil and I know that they've saved a LOT of lives. I am thankful for many things that the medical world has afforded us. But my good friend put it best when she said, "we aren't living longer... we are just dying slower". And it's so true.

What's interesting is that this rate of declining health has nearly matched the rate of increase of chemicals and synthetic products used in our society.

Our cleaning cabinets have gotten more complicated. Our bathroom cabinets and drawers now have all kinds of synthetic fragrances and man-made alternatives to natural bath, body and beauty remedies.

Our food supply has been depleted of minerals and vitamins because of overworked soil, made toxic by added chemicals, and is raising many unanswered questions on the safety of genetic modification. Every room in our house is inundated with toxins. And then we wonder why we aren't healthier. Guys, this history matters.

My Decision Based on Facts

Ok... let's recap. Here are the high points:
- I grew up involved in an agricultural home.
- I was inundated by and heavily studied the Ag industry in college.
- I married a man and his children who lost their wife and mom from

breast cancer at age 35.

- I had emotional baggage and many pregnancy losses.
- Then a miracle baby.
- Then a pursuit of a healthier life and my introduction to essential oils.
- And a 9 month crash course on natural living, clean eating, essential oils and meshing all of my past and present studies together.
- Finally, my decision to pursue *true* wellness.

… So where does this leave us? What I was realizing was that I truly do love nature. But what I thought was "natural" and "healthy" was *anything but* natural and healthy!

I attribute much of this new awareness to the company of essential oils I was using and studying.

Young Living Essential Oils officially launched in 1994, but Gary Young, its founder, had studied oils, natural medicine, and health & wellness for decades before that.

The integrity of Young Living's products, particularly their Seed to Seal standard—which I'll address in the next chapter—completely impressed me.

I thought back to when I was in high school and gave a presentation to elementary students called "From the Farm to the Table". It was a walk-through of the many steps it takes to get your food from a field in Nebraska to a dinner table in New Jersey. The steps were long and many.

It dawned on me that every company in the world has multiple vendors who "touch" their products during its stages from raw ingredients to the final product sold on store shelves. Every single company does this… unless you're shopping at a Farmer's Market and buying tomatoes grown in your neighbor's garden. This is one of a very few exceptions.

But with every other product we buy, each vendor has their bottom line in mind. They want to minimize expenses and maximize profits. That means that at any step of the process during the life of these products, someone could have cut a corner, used a lesser ingredient, or processed in a "more efficient" (but less natural) way in order to afford themselves the most profit possible.

This is basic business, it doesn't mean that these people are all bad… it's just the nature of the beast, and unfortunately, the consumers are the ones who suffer from these business decisions.

So, really... think about this... what did you eat this morning? Do you know what the life of that food has been? Probably not all of it...

What about what you're wearing... do you know where those fibers came from (if it's cotton)... or where the synthetic fibers were created?

And your shampoo you used in your last shower? Do you have any clue what makes up that liquid you squeeze into your wet hand?

And why does any of this information even matter?

It matters because my husband sat next to a hospital bed and said good-bye to the mother of his five children.

It matters because there are over 6,300 hospitals full of sick people across this country.

It matters because today, there are more people overweight in America than there are people who are a healthy weight.

Imagine the wheels of your car driving over hot, wet tar on a summer day... it completely gums up the wheels until they're a sticky, gooey mess. That is the mental picture I get when I think of adding toxic ingredients and chemicals to my natural body.

My cells want to BREATHE! Your cells want to BREATHE! They want life, vitality, oxygen, blood flow, and freedom to do what they were created to do.

Why do we think that we can add man-made chemical compounds to our systems by spraying things around us and breathing it in, rubbing and spraying things on our skin and hair, and eating or drinking things and then hoping that it won't ever affect us?

That doesn't even make sense. That's like saying, "ohhhh, I can TOTALLY eat cookies in front of the T.V. all day every day and never gain weight..." It's like math. 2 + 2 = 4. And no matter how much we want it to equal five, it just doesn't.

Our bodies are the same way. Science has proven that when you apply or use things in, on or around your body, those substances WILL enter your blood stream. Many of these ingredients will cross the blood-brain barrier or the placental barrier. Then our body has to try to recognize them, deal with them, and continue thriving.

Our bodies are amazing… they want to survive at all cost. We have a mental will to live, but a physical will to live as well. God gave us natural defense mechanisms. Adrenaline allows us to fight or flight when faced with danger. White blood cells fight off infections when we get sick. Our blood, liver, and various organs cleanse and filter much of the junk we are exposed to. God gave us an extra measure of grace to be exposed to harsh or dangerous things and still survive.

But we've pushed that limit too far. Just like one cookie won't cause you to be overweight, a little bit of "non-natural" products used on your body won't kill you. Still, everything has a threshold. Like the Jenga game I play with my kids… you can pull out some foundational pieces that are needed to hold the Jenga structure together time and time again… but at some point, one of those pieces is the final straw and the structure collapses.

Our bodies are similar to this. Yes, we have an extra measure of grace built in to deal with a harsh world… but why push it to the max and toe up to the line? I, for one, have never felt better than I have since I began pursuing a lifestyle of true health. (That doesn't necessarily mean hitting the pavement at 6am every day, either. Though I do think that an active lifestyle is important to overall health, our culture has led us to believe exercise IS wellness… but that sells short the concept of complete health).

Health and wellness is recognizing that our body can't be segmented off into parts. It all works together—emotionally, spiritually and physically. Also within our bodies, the organs work together, the major body systems work together, many parts are dependent on one another. If something goes wrong in one body system it could be because something in another system is off or somehow not functioning properly.

I am so done with this culture of sickness, aren't you? I am excited about pursuing health for myself and my family. I'm inspired to prevent my kids from losing another mom through every decision we make in our house. Seriously, it's our daily reality. I'm totally committed to preventing in them early onset issues like their birth mom dealt with.

I'm ready to rock this wellness thing. #CanIGetAnAmen

Chapter 2

Young Living:
The Perfect Addition to my Wellness Toolbox

I don't know about you, but I don't necessarily want to go back to the 1800's and mill our flour and make our lye soap for survival. But there has to be a happy medium—a daily, boots on the ground reality where modern sophistication and culture can still allow room for getting back to natural, basic, simple concepts and creations.

So, to get back to the basics in our home, we have tried to clean up all the areas of our lives where we put things in, on or around our bodies. We started in our kitchen. Here are a few good tips we learned that turned this mountain into a mole hill.

Our family is trying to eat foods as raw, real and whole as possible. This means fewer processed foods (fewer boxes, bags and cans); fewer refined sugars (store bought desserts and candy); and fewer empty carbs (breads, cereals and chips).

This also means more raw foods, particularly organic produce. (If you can't buy everything organic, google the dirty dozen); more real, good fats. (We don't ever eat fat free or sugar free. We eat real butter, whole milk, avocadoes, lots of nuts, etc.); and we go with natural sweeteners (raw, locally raised honey, coconut sugar, stevia or Blue Agave). We now make homemade breads or desserts with real ingredients. Our meals are simpler foods with fewer steps. And of course we love food from our garden, our chickens, farmer's markets, or locally sourced.

For much of the other consumable products in our home, we have traded synthetic for natural. Enter: *Young Living.*

This company has the best all natural, oil-infused products and the best essential oils on the planet.

They are truly a product-driven company (not a bottom-line drive company). And what's more: their standards aren't just words on a website… the way this company runs, and the foundation on which it's built is solid, genuine, and noble. *Their actions speak louder than their words.*

When I started using Young Living Essential Oils, I started to think more. I thought about labels of products in my house. I thought of my children's health. I thought about the agriculture industry differently. It truly opened my eyes to the world around us.

Today, I am inundated with the Young Living lifestyle… and it's not just because I have their products in every room of my home. It's also because I can look to this company as a role-model of sorts for my own lifestyle. They are truly people on a mission.

The Mission Statement

"We honor our stewardship to champion nature's living energy, essential oils, by fostering a community of healing and discovery while inspiring individuals to wellness, purpose, and abundance."

– Young Living Essential Oils Mission Statement[2]

The neat thing about this mission statement is that each word is carefully chosen to represent to the world who Young Living is.

This is truly the Young Living difference and why this company, founded and owned by a farmer and his wife, is so impressive.

They have beautiful, whole, clean products… yet they're the best kept secret in the world.

Young Living's product line is only getting more solid, effective, and health-focused. They cut no corner and spare no expense. Let's break this mission statement down to get to the heart of who Young Living is. #TheyAreTheRealDeal

Stewardship

Young Living all about stewardship, which means protecting and being responsible for something. They recognize that this lost art of distilling plants to extract their oils is a delicate and important process. Young Living understands how essential oils are one of God's gifts to humanity. They can't be rushed, manipulated, or seen as just tools for profit. They are a part of our total health… and if they are produced properly, they provide enormous benefits to those who use them—even the missing link in our wellness.

What does Young Living do to steward these plants, oils, and oil-infused products so meticulously? It's what sets them apart from every other health company in the world and it's called their Seed to Seal guarantee. They describe it as:

*We diligently scrutinize every step of our production process to bring you the purest products the earth has to offer. We call it... **Seed to Seal**. It's not a slogan—it's our calling.*[3]

The seed to seal process includes the many steps of production that most companies around the world broker out.

Young Living started with Gary Young producing his first 3ml bottle of lavender oil that was grown on his own farm and distilled in his own small, hand built distillery. Then he studied the oil and its chemical constituents and used the oil himself.

From there, Gary and Mary Young have bought and cultivated farms around the world. Today Young Living owns thousands of acres of farmland worldwide and they also have thousands of acres of partner farms, where they employ local experts and they have full governance of that property. Here's a quick overview of the Seed to Seal process:

Seed: On the farms, before planting the seeds, Young Living ensures that the soil has the proper pH, that it's organic in nature, and that the soil composition is ideal for the plants that will be grown there. They plant their seeds, many of which are collected from the best, most vigorous plants of the previous growing season.

Cultivate: Once the seeds are planted, Young Living cultivates and grows the plants *beyond* organically. They don't add pesticides, fertilizers and other chemicals. Well trained and passionate workers tend to the plants as a master gardener would meticulously tend to his garden. No detail goes unnoticed.

As we know, organic food is more expensive because it is way more labor intensive and requires smaller batches and more attention. Young Living's oils are no different. They have increased their footprint from one tiny farm to thousands of acres around the world and have taught, trained and implemented the same production practices with the local experts and workers at every single property and distillery.

Once the plant, tree, or flower is at peak performance in its life cycle, it is harvested with appropriate methods for maximizing the quality of the oil. Sometimes this includes harvesting a flower during early morning hours. Other times this means the harvest window is only a few weeks out of the whole year in order to best protect the plant and its oil.

If an essential oil company has no say in these important steps, there's no way of knowing how cultivation and harvest were conducted. Understand that that tiny molecule of oil is in the plant from the beginning—it's up to the steward of that molecule to protect it during each step of this process.

Distill: The parts of the plant that are used for oil production (which might be the leaves, stems, roots, flowers, or bark) are added to a big metal vat—some holding thousands of pounds of plant matter—and then steam is pushed up from the bottom through the plant materials, condensing at the top. This liquid is separated between the floral water and the essential oil.

Basic chemistry tells us that when you apply heat and pressure to a substance, the chemical composition of that substance changes. This process of distillation is critical. If too much or not enough heat or pressure are added for too long or too short of a time, it can change that oil into something much less valuable and effective, even harmful. This process is PARAMOUNT!

Gary Young and his team have built every distillery right on their farms and they've worked to perfect the process over the past two decades.

Test: The next step is testing. Young Living only keeps oils that meet certain chemical constituent requirements. They test each and every batch, and then do additional testing that is above and beyond international industry standards, including third party testing. What's more, they don't add hidden preservatives, fillers, additives, or carriers to stretch out the oil.

Seal: Young Living's goal is not to produce as much oil as possible, but rather that each batch is perfect and whole and will provide value to the person using it. (I love this because it makes it so personal to my bottles of oils sitting around on my bathroom and kitchen counters).

Young Living represents true love and stewardship of essential oils… and this passion is something that no other company can parallel.

When Vince Lombardi was the coach of the Green Bay Packers professional football team he said, "The harder you work, the harder it is to surrender." This quote embodies is why Young Living takes every meticulous detail seriously. They work so hard to produce perfection every time—so they surrender no detail for convenience, cost savings, or ease.

This is a calling that Young Living believes is genuinely changing people's lives. (It's changed mine!)

So when you break that seal to use their products, take a deep breath and be grateful for a company that cares about your health and the health of your family nearly as much as you do!

Young Living inspires us to be better because we only have one body and one life to live. We don't get to do whatever we want and then hit the backspace button and do it over again. What we put in, on and around ourselves truly does have an effect on our organs, our systems, and our overall health.

If Young Living goes to such great lengths to take care of the small details—because they matter—how much more should we consider every chemical and every toxin and make choices to be good stewards of our own bodies?

Champion

Championing something is to be excellent in that area. The Young's lead a company of excellence—from their Seed to Seal process, to the choices they make in business, to their customer service, to their executive team. This company is all about excellence in every way.

I heard Gary tell a neat story on a phone call one time. He was in Canada, at the Northern Lights farm they had just purchased. It was winter, and about 50 degrees below zero, yet they worked straight through because Young Living members needed Back Spruce, and Valor—one of the most popular oil blends which contains Black Spruce. Gary was there the whole time, barely breaking for Christmas, working on the tractors, helping map out plans for the distillery, and so on.

The Canadian government had implemented a new regulation in recent years because a boiler had exploded at another company's work site and badly injured people. This incident mandated that the water meet certain requirements for all new boilers built. (And boilers are a very important aspect of a distillery).

In order to be compliant, most companies added a tank with chemicals that the water could filter through in order to meet that requirement. Well, Young Living doesn't operate with synthetic, harsh chemicals... so instead of doing this quick and easy step—they made the choice to be a company of excellence and instead built an *entire water treatment plant right on the farm*.

Umm, wow. That is excellence in the raw. This story totally impressed me. It made me love Young Living so much more. Something like this would be great for marketing to the world what they do. They could have solidified so many loyal oil users by this story, increasing their territory and their customer base. But they don't blast their "good deeds" all over the place, because it is just who they are—their core is genuine and real. When you are genuine and real about what you believe, there is not even a choice to make… you simply do the right thing.

I am continually learning new pieces of amazing information about Young Living—and any one of them could make for a great article, and yet I'm never surprised at the level of integrity this company shows and the commitment to championing everything they do.

For my family, and for me, Young Living inspires us towards being a champion of our own lives. This means commitment to excellence with all the hats we wear. It's being the best 'you' possible! For me, that means being the best I can be as a Christian, wife, mom, friend and health coach.

Being involved with Young Living not only means using the best products in the world, which help me towards excellence because I have the energy, focus and stamina to do them… but it also means working with a company who is truly like iron sharpening iron… where I'm constantly looking at the integrity Young Living has and wanting to live that out in my own life.

Community

This company embraces community. The communities where they have their farms, the friendships at the corporate offices, and the entire Young Living family of members.

Young Living is a company of people who are all about other people. One of my favorite stories of how Young Living embraces the concept of community is that they are the only essential oil company in the world allowed to work in the Middle Eastern country of Oman with their ancient Sacred Frankincense trees.

Other companies have been asked to leave or not let in in the first place because they have profit of the forefront of their mind. On the contrary, what Young Living does is honor the age-old traditions and customs of those tribes who've been harvesting Frankincense resin for thousands of years.

When Young Living came into Oman, Gary worked closely with the officials and locals to cultivate a relationship of integrity.

The Sacred Frankincense trees are raised and the resin is harvested by families who have lived in those communities since Biblical times! These community members know exactly how to extract it from the trees in a way that is the most potent for the oil and the most sustainable for the tree.

Young Living built a distillery on the Frankincense farm in Oman and they have a fabulous working relationship with the people there.

Also, the Young Living Foundation is supporting people in underprivileged communities around the world. For example, the Foundation supports a school in Ecuador and works with families and children in Africa helping them implement healthy living practices. Young Living members and leaders contribute to the Foundation to support all that Young Living does worldwide.

Another element of community that Young Living has embraced is understanding that balance is key. So they partnered with an awesome company called Oola because Oola is "changing the world with a word". This word Oola (from the idea of oo-la-la) is all about being balanced in these seven areas of your life: Family, Friends, Faith, Fitness, Fun, Finance and Field—which in turn help strengthen your own community.

Individuals

Young Living is a company of members that does everything for the individual. When Gary stays up until two in the morning watching a new oil being distilled, he does that with YOU in mind. He cares, and the company cares, about the individual person. He knows that when you open your personal bottles of oils or oil-infused products, that you're using it to support your body or your children's bodies... and that is important!

The ways that Young Living empowers me as an individual is the reason I really embraced my freedom of choice as a wife, mom and person. I realized the truth in what my dad had been teaching me all my life—which is that we are an individual, with independent thought and self-governed choice making ability. We do not have to do what is mainstream just because it's mainstream.

We can think outside the box, be a problem solver, and seek out effective solutions that are better and healthier!

Young Living gives us the option to not conform to this world. As a company they recognize that God gave us the dignity of choice. First demonstrated in our ability to choose Him, and then every other decision we make as well.

Wellness

Woo Hoo! You know what? Young Living is a wellness company! Everything they do is about helping us be totally healthy!!!

The coolest part of this is that it's totally NOT just an overused catch phrase. Health and wellness is at the core of Young Living, *because they get it.*

They understand that the body isn't overly complicated. If you add toxins to it, it doesn't work right... plain and simple. If you use oils and oil-infused products that penetrate to the cellular level to pull toxins out, then you will just be healthier! Things in your body... functions, systems... they just work better. Period.

I love this because I want to be focused on my health and wellness and that of my family! Don't you?

Not adding toxic chemicals is the primary reason we use Young Living's products because their seal guarantees a "good for you" product that is infused with their amazing Seed to Seal essential oils. The oils can help our bodies cleanse and detox and many of them support major functions and systems that make us "go"! (Because the home products are oil-infused they have an added advantage over the more natural products we can get on the store shelves). This is the Young Living difference.

Young Living is all about helping you and I be WELL, today, tomorrow, and the rest of our lives!

#omgoodness #SoAwesome #RevOILution

Purpose

Young Living is a purpose driven company. Their purpose is to get essential oils and oil-infused products into every home in the world. Everything they do is toward that end.

When they buy farms, produce oils, host educational and recognition events, research new plants around the world, employ thousands of people, and support millions of members... it is all for creating a movement of wellness across the globe and utilizing their incredible product line to do it!

In our lives, we really need to have a bigger purpose than just going with the flow every day. If you aren't moving forward, you're moving backwards. Be intentional. Be on purpose... don't wait for everything to happen and take a "wait and see" stance. Young Living creates a purpose driven culture.

Abundance

Abundance means overflow, excess, more than enough. Young Living creates abundance in all that they do because of their stewardship of producing the best essential oils; championing every area; their respect for communities and empowering of individuals; having a heart and soul for health and wellness; and being a purpose driven company. Young Living is all about overflow of all things good.

When I think of overflow for our lives, I am so blessed that we have found abundance in Young Living. Our health, our relationships with other health-minded friends, our finances, our freedom to give, and our opportunities to bless and educate others on their own journey have all come from Young Living.

Write Your Own Mission Statement

More often than not, people who start using Young Living products are just normal, everyday folks who are pretty much *not* complete health and wellness gurus.

It's only once people begin seeing how amazing the oils and oil-infused products are that they start to try to be healthy in other areas... because choosing products that are awesome is a little addicting.

When we start to realize our value as a person, and we are inspired by a company that doesn't just treat us like a number, it's easy to want to be excellent. People matter. Mission statements matter.

What's your mission statement? Could you use Young Living's as a model for your own life, your family, your marriage, your business, and at the core of who you are?

Think about what mission you want to live out. Then write it down. Then look at it again tomorrow. Modify, edit, adapt. Think about it again. Share it with someone else. Have a plan and a purpose.

You're awesome. #TheYoungLivingLifestyleRocks

Chapter 3:

A Day in the Life of...

So we get that Young Living does things the right way. We can tremendously benefit from the products they provide as well as the character of the company that we can use as a role model for our own lives. What would it look like to incorporate Young Living products into your everyday life?

In this chapter, you will see the many oils and oil-infused products that Young Living leaders use. Many of them have made a career of educating people on the Young Living lifestyle.

When you think of changing over the toxic, chemically-laden stuff in your house, it can be overwhelming. I hear you!

Just take a look at some of these leaders' daily lives. Some of them have been using wellness products for decades, others just for a year or less. But every single person is absolutely in LOVE with Young Living.

Note the variation in age, gender, interests, and regions of the country (even a few from around the world—as Young Living has a significant global community). Also, read "What does Young Living mean to you?" for each leader. We are living out the Young Living Lifestyle and are changing the world, one drop of oil at a time. Join us! Your health matters. #WeLoveYou.

Adam Green

Royal Crown Diamond, Canada

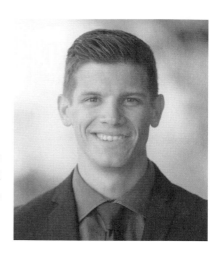

YL member since? 2007

Spouse: Vanessa Green

Age: 26

Hobbies: Skiing, skydiving, traveling, public speaking, lake activities... anything for a good adrenaline rush! Also writing! (See my site www.25toLifeBook.com for details.)

Favorite Young Living product? NingXia Red & Nitro

Favorite Young Living farm or event? Annual Leadership Cruise

Describe your day using Young Living products:

Morning: Lavender Mint shampoo and conditioner, Morning Start body wash, ART Skin Care System, Thieves, Valor, Super B, True Source, OmegaGize3, Longevity, NingXia Red, NingXia Nitro, mixed with sparkling water (NingXia Spritzer), Sulfurzyme capsules, one of the Young Living shakes, and Essentialzyme-4's

Afternoon: Essentialzyme-4's, MultiGreens, Peppermint

Evening: Life 5, Sulfurzyme, OmegaGize3, ImmuPro, Peace & Calming, Tranquil, RutaVaLa, Cedarwood, Lavender, diffuse oils.

When Traveling: Everyday Oils Kit, Cedarwood, travel diffuser, ImmuPro, Core Supplements, NingXia Red & Nitro

What does Young Living mean to you?

Young Living is about helping others develop their best physical and financial health. It's empowering others to live their true calling in life, while living a life of purpose and influence. I can't picture myself doing anything else. Every day I wake up grateful for the opportunity to create change in the lives of thousands of people.

What is your favorite clean eating meal? Anything ethnic... I really love Thai Food, salad rolls, etc.

Alina Rinato

Platinum, Florida

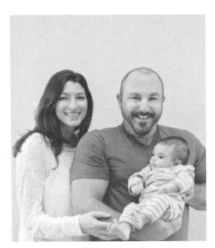

YL member since? 2009
Spouse: Rob Rinato
Age: 32
Hobbies: Travel, beach days, boating, playing with our son, collecting Young Living oils
Favorite Young Living product? Neroli
Favorite Product to Gift? Everyday Oils

Favorite Young Living farm or event? Master Leader Retreat at the Ecuador farm

Describe your day using Young Living products:

Morning: Diffuse Citrus Fresh + Abundance, NingXia Red, MultiGreens, enzymes, Sulfurzyme, Thieves toothpaste, Lavender shampoo, Morning Start bath gel, Orange Blossom face wash, Satin Mint face scrub, ART face moisturizer. Apply Progessence Plus, and eat a fruit smoothie with Balance Complete

Afternoon: Diffuse Frankincense, drink more NingXia Red or Nitro if needed. Lavender for nap time for Roman, Peppermint or Clarity if working in the office.

Evening: NingXia Red spritzer with dinner (a La Croix drink or allergen water with 2 ounces NingXia Red and 2 drops of Grapefruit or Tangerine oils), Lavender and Cedarwood in the diffuser and applied for bedtime, ART cleanser, toner, moisturizer, Thieves toothpaste, Thieves floss, Multi Greens, Life 5, enzymes, and Sulfurzyme before bed.

When Traveling: DiGize, Peppermint, Lavender, Lemon, Bon Voyage kit, Thieves hand purifier, NingXia Red and Nitro

What does Young Living mean to you? In one word, Young Living means *lifestyle* for us. It allows us to build a business based on our values. It has given us the time freedom to be stay at home parents while we work together to help others realize their dreams of Wellness, Purpose and Abundance.

What is your favorite clean eating meal? Grilled shrimp over organic greens with Lemon essential oil, vinaigrette, goat cheese, walnuts, dried cranberries and clementine slices!

Amanda Uribe
Diamond, Alaska

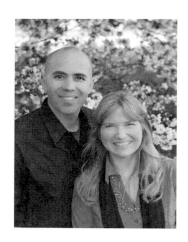

YL member since? 2013

Spouse: Gabe Uribe

Age: 39

Hobbies: Avid reader, homeschool mom. I love cooking, hanging with my family outdoors, camping and exploring.

Favorite Young Living product?
Frankincense & BLM

Favorite Product to Gift? NingXia

Favorite Young Living farm or event? The Ecuador farm

Describe **your day using Young Living products:**

Morning: Supplements: BLM, Essentialzyme, Master Formula, Prenolone cream. Oils: I love to use Frankincense, Lemon, Endoflex, sometimes Grapefruit or Thieves. Oils topically include Frankincense, Lavender, Purification on face for healthy skin tone. I love to use Peppermint to wake up. Peppermint and Cinnamon oil in coffee. Stress away for the day ahead.

Afternoon: Slique tea, Slique gum, Slique Bar, MultiGreens, Lemon oil in water, Super C, Super B, BLM, ComforTone, Digest + Cleanse. What I apply topically depends on the day. Harmony, Highest Potential, Release, En-R-Gee, Dragon Time, Progessence Plus, Valor, PanAway, Lavender, Thieves, Deep Relief... It really just depends on what is going on that day.

Evening: BLM, ComforTone. Sulfurzyme, ART skincare system, Sheerlumé Brightening Cream and Ortho Sport. Oils: Idaho Balsam Fir, Lemongrass, Valor, Wintergreen, Oregano, Copaiba, Peace & Calming, Thieves.

When Traveling: All of the above plus all of the Juva products & more Essentialzymes.

What does Young Living mean to you? Family. Our family of four has grown several thousand times bigger because we joined Young Living. Between farm events, conventions, rank clubs and grand openings around the world, we have had the amazing opportunity to meet and really get to know so many phenomenal people who have become family. What we find so amazing is that it isn't just about Young Living. Sure, that is where our core lies. Really, though, it is about living well and to our fullest potential. We all share commonality in food, health, and lifestyle choices and a desire to live in wellness through the use of essential oils.

Andrew Jenkins
Platinum, Alabama

Young Living member since? 2013
Spouse: Cristy Jenkins
Age: 41
Children: 9 (Ages 2 to 14)
Hobbies: Running, cross training, writing, reading.
Favorite Young Living product? Power Meal. I used this last spring when I was losing weight. I still use it daily.

Favorite Young Living farm or event?
Drive to Win, Hawaiian Sandalwood Farm

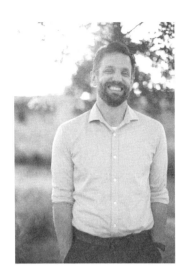

Describe your day using Young Living products:

Morning: Brush with Thieves toothpaste. Power Meal, Idaho Blue Spruce—5 drops in a shot of NingXia Red, Cedarwood on my head, Shutran on my wrists, neck and beard (if I have one at the time), Bath Gel—unscented. (I mix Shutran with it.) Mint deodorant, DiGize, Master Formula, MultiGreens, Longevity. Sometimes for kids: NingXia Red with Thieves. I sometimes roll Valor on a leather bracelet.

Afternoon: DiGize on the tongue, Lemon in water.

Evening: Brush with Thieves toothpaste, DiGize on the tongue, MultiGreens. Sometimes I sleep with the use of the Freedom Sleep kit. We often tuck our kids into bed with Lavender and/or Peace & Calming.

When Traveling: Same as above. We take the products with us in smaller containers.

What does Young Living mean to you? Young Living has provided a venue for us to walk in health and wholeness with more success than we've ever had. We've met incredible friends and we've been blessed financially as our team has grown. We've also found an opportunity to work together as a team in a unique way, bringing simplicity to our lives while walking in abundance.

What is your favorite clean eating meal? Filet Mignon, brown rice, salad and hummus.

April Pointer
Royal Crown Diamond, Texas

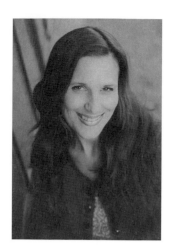

Young Living member since? 2009

Spouse: Jay Pointer

Age: 40

Hobbies: Soap making, travel, laser tag with my boys & working out. Favorite things are my home state (Texas!), the mountains, family walks, kombucha, Mexican food and cats.

Favorite Young Living product? DiGize and Believe oil blends and Multi Greens and Sulfurzyme

Favorite Young Living farm or event? Gold Retreat in Ecuador in 2013 and Young Living Cruise in 2015

Describe your day using Young Living products:

I like to get our supplements in at least 4-5 days a week and love that they're full of so many nutrients that I can skips days here and there. My supply last longer this way too. My family uses NingXia Red, MultiGreens, Sulfurzyme, Orange or Cinnamon in NingXia, Apply frankincense to my face with a little bit of Rose oil or Sandalwood 2-3 times a week. We like to diffuse oils that wake us up like Purification or Eucalyptus with other oils as a blend. My kids love Stress Away and Wintergreen in the diffuser, it smells like a root beer float! Baths with Stress away, Sacred Mountain or Lavender are a hit! I like Valor as a facial moisturizer.

When Traveling: Immune boosting oils along with Peppermint, DiGize, Lemon and Valor. ComforTone, MultiGreens, Detoxzyme. I take BLM and Sulfurzyme just in case.

What does Young Living mean to you? Young Living was the missing link for my family. We were already a holistic family but were missing QUALITY essential oils. It has been a life changing journey for my family. Not only have we been able to optimize our family's health with it but God has called us to inspire change in the world through natural health. At Royal Crown Diamond, our dream is being fulfilled in being able to financially contribute generously to ministries and organizations my husband and I are passionate about. Young Living gives every member the platform to share health and wellness without compromise because our products work and we operate with utmost integrity. My favorite thing is that Young Living is for EVERYONE and we are thriving because Young Living rewards us for sharing what we love.

Ashley McKenney
Diamond, Florida

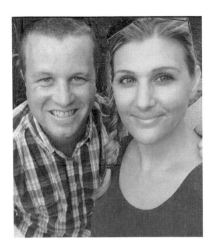

YL member since? 2013

Spouse: Ryan McKenney

Age: 31

Hobbies: Reading, writing, photography, beach combing

Favorite Young Living product? Eucalyptus Radiata because it makes the room an instant spa

Favorite Product to Gift? Anything Thieves

Favorite Young Living farm or event? THRIVE has been my favorite. I loved the speakers and adored staying at the Gaylord Opry Resort.

Describe your day using Young Living products:

Morning: Brush my teeth with Thieves toothpaste and Orange oil. Swipe on some rose ointment while I drink coffee/wake up. Make a NingXia Red smoothie, followed by a Nitro shot.

Afternoon: I diffuse Eucalyptus, Sandalwood and Cedarwood throughout the house to promote a relaxing atmosphere. After nap, I take another shot of Nitro.

Evening: Brush teeth with Thieves toothpaste & Orange oil. Wash face with Orange facial scrub, apply Rose Ointment all over face. Use Purification and Frankincense for problem areas. Pick my good night diffusing combo and apply oils for some good rest... it's different every night. I love trying new combinations.

When Traveling: Depending on the day and situation I could take different things. I load up on Inner Defense and MultiGreens. Even when traveling, the morning, afternoon and night routine is pretty solid.

What does Young Living mean to you? Young Living means financial freedom. It means living our lives in the healthiest way possible. Promoting wellness in every cell structure and function. Young Living means time with my family. It means meeting new people, helping those who would like to venture into the world of natural health. Honestly, Young Living equals living out our dreams.

Becky Webb

Diamond, North Carolina

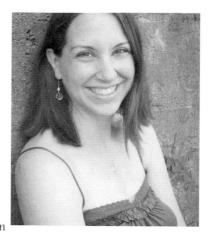

Young Living member since? 2013

Spouse: Jonathan Webb

Age: 34

Hobbies: Reading, learning, pampering and self-care after years of not being able to.

Favorite Young Living product?
Thieves Cleaner

Favorite Young Living farm or event? 2015 Global Leadership Cruise to the Mediterranean

Describe your day using Young Living products:

Morning: Diffuse Lemon and Peppermint oil to get us going. I add a drop or two of Lemon to my breakfast shake. Then the whole family will take shots of NingXia Red. I apply Jasmine over my heart and Envision on my temples to help with feeling overwhelmed. Morning and night I LOVE the Thieves AromaBright toothpaste! My teeth are sparkling! I will also apply Endoflex over my thyroid and adrenals in the morning from a roller ball. In the shower I will use the Lavender Mint shampoo.

Afternoon: I use Carrot Seed and Lavender oil in a homemade lotion that we use before swimming. We also use some grapefruit lip balm post-swimming. After coming home, we diffuse some Valor to get some good relaxation time at home.

Evening: I love to use oils like Basil, Thyme, Lemon and Oregano for cooking. I made green beans the other day with some Lemon and Basil. Delicious! Or Peppermint brownies for desert! Yummy! After dinner I use the Thieves cleaner to wipe down my counters and the table. Every evening my kids will ask for their oils at bed time. I'll use SleepyIze, Cedarwood or Lavender to help encourage a restful sleep. I use the Thieves mouthwash and toothpaste.

What does Young Living mean to you? Young Living has been an incredible blessing for our family. I'm passionate about seeing people healthy and with Young Living I am able to share products that do exactly that! Young Living enabled my husband to leave a job where he had to be gone for more than 70 days a year. He can now be home all the time and continually invest in the lives of his children. We love the freedom to pursue what we love.

Callie Shepherd
Crown Diamond, Oklahoma

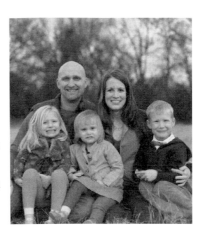

Young Living member since? 2012

Spouse: Jeremy Shepherd

Age: 33

Hobbies: Graphic design, hiking, sipping a hot cup of Scottish Breakfast

Favorite Young Living product? NingXia Red

Favorite Young Living product gift? NingXia Nitro

Favorite Young Living farm or event?

Describe your day using Young Living products:

Morning: Rise and Shine! Start our day with NingXia Red, AromaBright toothpaste (which doubles as deodorant!) then Essentialzyme and MultiGreens, Sacred Mountain + Peppermint going in the diffuser, I often grab Valor before chiropractor appointment and grab Ortho Ease to take with me to my massage.

Afternoon: NingXia + afternoon shot of Nitro + tablespoon of MindWise and often Owie and Lavender oils for the kids.

Evening: Time for dinner and more Essentialzyme + MightyZyme. At bedtime, Cedarwood in the kids diffuser, ImmuPower on their feet. My evening beauty routine – ART Cleanser + Satin Mint Facial Scrub + ART moisturizer with a drop of Elemi essential oil and wind down with Stress Away on neck and temples, and Peace & Calming on feet.

When Traveling: Thieves lozenges + Essentialzyme + lots of water for airplane + Nitro + SleepEssence to manage jetlag. Clove oil + empty vegetable capsules to boost immune system while traveling + AromaEase for any digestive soothing. Deep Relief to sooth minor head tension, Lemon for all foreign water. NingXia Red + Slique Bars for overall energy during hectic times and when meals are hard to come by.

What does Young Living mean to you? Young Living has become an anchor in our lives as we look to the products daily for our overall health and wellness. Also, the community of likeminded oilers around us has created friendships and relationships that will last a lifetime.

Camille Seever
Gold, Missouri

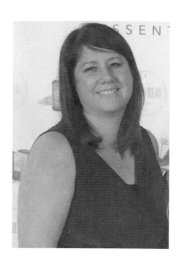

Young Living member since? 2013
Spouse: Brent Seever
Age: 44
Hobbies: Homeschooling, singing
Favorite Young Living product? Abundance, Fennel, Progessence Plus
Favorite Young Living product gift? Whatever I feel led at the time.
Favorite Young Living farm or event? The Mona Farm. It's so family friendly.

Describe your day using Young Living products:

Morning: Thieves AromaBright toothpaste and mouthwash, Copaiba Vanilla shampoo, Morning Start shower gel, ART Gentle Cleanser, ART Renewal Serum, ART Light Moisturizer, Mountain Mint Deodorant, Genesis or Sensation lotion, MindWise, Ning-Xia Red, Digest + Cleanse, Master Formula, OmegaGize, and Progessence Plus.

Afternoon: Nitro, Slique Tea and various oils like Slique Essence, Abundance, Awaken, Highest Potential, Frankincense and White Angelica.

Evening: Thyromin, Grapefruit oil

When Traveling: AromaBright toothpaste, Thieves mouthwash, Copaiba Vanilla shampoo, Morning Start Shower Gel, ART Gentle Cleanser, ART Renewal Serum, ART Light Moisturizer, Mountain Mint Deodorant, Genesis or Sensation Hand and Body Lotion, NingXia Red, Nitro and Progessence Plus.

What does Young Living mean to you? So Young Living means a ton to me. I don't know where I would have been without Young Living when Caden was born. The drug exposure caused such digestive discomfort for him. His digestive system is so much better since using DiGize regularly. And since drug exposed babies often have cognitive issues in addition to digestive issues we have been working on Young Living products that support cognitive development and he is doing amazing so far! They bring hope to so many.

What is your favorite clean eating meal? Grass-fed lamb chops, rice & asparagus.

Carla Green
Diamond, Canada

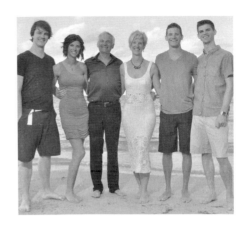

Young Living member since? 2000
Spouse: Bill Green
Age: 57
Hobbies: Reading, traveling, dancing, healthy living, gardening, hiking, teaching through secondchanceface.com
Favorite Young Living product?
Everyday Oils kit

Favorite Young Living product gift? Deep Relief roll on

Favorite Young Living farm or event? Global Leadership Cruise 2007

Describe your day using Young Living products:
Morning: ART foaming face wash, ART toner, ART Renewal Serum, Sheerlumé, Copaiba Vanilla shampoo and conditioner, Thieves toothpaste, mouthwash, dental floss, foaming hand soap, Young Living Bar Soap, Sulfurzyme, OmegaGize3, NingXia Red, Essentialzymes-4, GLF, Orange oil, Frankincense. Oil for diffuser (changes daily). Progessence Phyto Plus, EndoGize, adrenal and vision support blends.
Afternoon: Essentialzymes-4, NingXia, Thieves household cleaner & sanitizer.
Evening: ImmuPro, Sulfurzyme, Essentialzymes-4, OmegaGize3, Detoxzyme, Orange oil, adrenal support blend, vision support blend, Tranquil, RutaVaLa, Cedarwood.
When Traveling: Inner Defense, Everyday oils kit, Raindrop kit, Copaiba, Essentialzymes-4, Detoxzyme, ImmuPro, Longevity, Deep Relief, Tranquil, Breathe Again, DiGize, AromaEase, SleepEssence, Thieves hand sanitizer, Thieves spray, LavaDerm, ClaraDerm, Carrot Seed, Myrrh, Cedarwood and Lavender lotion.

What does Young Living mean to you? My passions are helping others achieve optimal health and preventing and reversing the signs of aging naturally. Young Living helps me to empower others to take charge of their own health. I LOVE having financially independent children that pay it forward. I LOVE the Young Living lifestyle, although that is the icing on the cake of helping people.

Carol Howden
Diamond, Canada

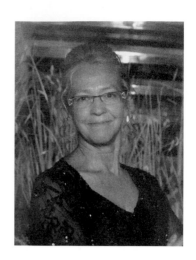

Young Living member since? 1999
Spouse: Ben Howden
Age: 60
Hobbies: Hiking, yachting
Favorite Young Living product? Valor
Favorite Young Living product gift?
Any oil from the Starter kit
Favorite Young Living farm or event?
Balsam Fir Harvest

Describe your day using Young Living products:

Morning: ComforTone, Thyromin, Mineral Essence, MindWise, Longevity, Aroma Life, Endoflex and En-R-Gee over the adrenals. I put NingXia Red into a large cup and fill it with hot water. Longevity capsules followed by shower with Lavender Mint shampoo and Morning Start shower gel. In my bathroom: Dentarome toothpaste, Thieves foaming hand soap, Ylang Ylang as deodorant. On face: Melrose followed with several drops of The Gift + Sheerlumé. I also apply Prenolone cream to my face and neck. I have two spritz bottles. Water with 10 drops of Abundance and Frankincense in one and 10 drops each of Acceptance and Frankincense. I take Essentialzyme and Super Cal. Then Super B, OmegaGize, MultiGreens, a capsule of DiGize and then every 30 minutes, I apply Endoflex over my thyroid and kidneys. At the same time I apply En-R-Gee.

Afternoon: Essentialzyme, Longevity and MultiGreens. At noon, I take 8-10 drops of DiGize with my meal. Mid-afternoon I take Longevity capsules.

Evening: Mineral Essence, MindWise. Then several drops of Melrose to my face followed with The Gift. Aroma Life, Goldenrod & Helichrysum over heart, Endoflex, SclarEssence, Australian Blue, Cypress, Idaho Blue Spruce, and Lavender topically, Valor and Joy on my feet, RutaVaLa on my neck.

What does Young Living mean to you? Young Living is a lifestyle where our short term and our long term goals are to manifest a life of wholeness, continuing to teach others how to enhance health and prosperity. We know we can do this through Young Living. It is a company we feel has the highest of standards; one that is committed to research in supplying solutions for health and longevity. Young Living is truly a company with integrity and vision.

Carol Yeh-Garner
Diamond, California

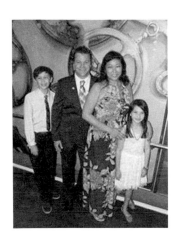

Young Living member since? 2013

Spouse: Scott Garner

Age: 45

Hobbies: Going to the beach, reading, hanging out with family and friends, traveling

Favorite Young Living product? Thieves oil because it's the oil that got me started

Favorite Young Living product gift? Thieves

Describe your day using Young Living products:

Morning: Brush with Thieves AromaBright toothpaste. Young Living shower gel with Frankincense and Lavender added to it. Mint facial scrub every other day. Genesis lotion after showering. Grapefruit lip balm. ART Light Moisturizer on my face. Joy over my heart and Humility on my wrists. NingXia Red packet as part of my breakfast. Lemon, Peppermint and Lavender as needed. Clarity, Master Formula, EndoGize.

Afternoon: Deep Relief on my neck after working at the. Diffuse various oils determined by my mood. Abundance and Build Your Dream on my wrists.

Evening: I diffuse various oils determined by my kids' moods. En-R-Gee to help me get through the rest of the day. I might use a drop of DiGize if I feel bloated. Before bed, I take Sulfurzyme and Life 5. Bedtime routine: Sheerlumé with a drop of Joy, Frankincense and Lavender on my face. Cedarwood massaged into my scalp. Progessence Plus and Endoflex on my neck. SclarEssence on my lower abdomen. Valor on my big toes before bedtime. Geranium on the sides of my feet. A mixture of Thieves and Tea Tree rolled onto the soles of my feet. Lavender or Cedarwood in the diffuser as we sleep. We also diffuse oil in the kids' rooms .

When Traveling: I bring my diffuser! I also bring Joy, Thieves, Purification, Cedarwood, Lavender, Frankincense, Lemon, Copaiba, Deep Relief, PanAway, Helichrysum, En-R-Gee, Motivation, Humility, Grounding, Digize, Valor and Stress Away. I always bring enough NingXia Red packets so I can have 1-2 per day. I also bring my travel size toiletries—toothpaste, shampoo, conditioner

What does Young Living mean to you? Young Living is a company that is dedicated to healthy living. They are committed to ensuring that only the most pure, truly 100% natural products are provided to us. I love that by using their products, my family & I can live a cleaner, healthier, more balanced life.

Chelle Carter
Diamond, Texas

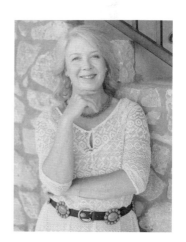

Young Living member since? 2004

Favorite Young Living product?
ART Renewal Serum

Favorite Young Living product gift? Thieves Spray

Favorite Young Living farm or event? The Highland Flats Farm

Describe your day using Young Living products:

Morning: Before I get out of bed, I grab an oil from my "Morning Box" which currently includes Awaken, Believe, Sacred Mountain, Transformation, Valor. Then Thieves toothpaste and mouthwash and the ART System and Sensation or Cel-Lite Magic Massage Oil. And I can't leave the bathroom without using the Young Living deodorant. I take Essentialzyme, Sulfurzyme, ComforTone, and CortiStop. Breakfast includes Power Meal, NingXia Red to my water bottle and White Angelica on each shoulder. Before lunch: Slique Slim Caps, MultiGreens, and Mineral Essence, and MindWise or OmegaGize.

Afternoon: Peppermint or Aroma Siez up and down my spine. I diffuse oils according to what we are doing and I always chew a piece of Slique Gum in the afternoon because I love the Frankincense Resin.

Evening: My favorite oils added to some Epsom salts for the bath are Joy, Lavender and Relieve It. In the shower, I alternate between the Lavender Mint and Copaiba Vanilla Shampoo/Conditioners. I shave using the conditioner as a shaving cream. My nighttime supplements Before bed, I choose favorite oils from my "Good Night Box" next to my bed. This includes Cedarwood, Peace & Calming, Frankincense and Lavender.

What does Young Living mean to you? Simplicity. Freedom. Hope. These compact, versatile, potent little oils minimize the clutter of multiple cabinets in my home and at the same time are easily used by every member of the family. Our homes are freed from the chemicals of this modern world, our bodies are freed from the burden of toxic overload, and thanks to the network marketing opportunity, our finances are freed from great strain. But, most of all, I value the hope that I see in people's eyes when they discover these great products.

Chelsea Flaman
Diamond, Canada

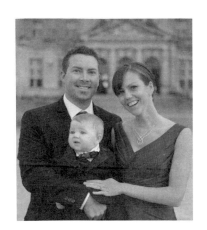

Young Living member since? 2012

Spouse: Jamie Flaman

Age: 30

Hobbies: Homeschooling, love to read & study scripture, knitting, crafts with kids

Favorite Young Living product? MultiGreens

Favorite Young Living product gift? Satin Mint scrub or DIY facial serum (Frankincense, Sandalwood and Rose in an avocado oil base).

Favorite Young Living farm or event? Croatia

Describe your day using Young Living products:

Morning: Dentarome Plus toothpaste, Thieves floss, Morning Start body wash, Lavender shampoo (my favorite shampoo by far for oily hair), Balance Complete, MindWise, NingXia, MultiGreens, Super B, Super C and Sulfurzyme. Skin care regime: ART Cleanser, ART Toner, homemade face serum, ART moisturizer.

Afternoon: Nitro and another shot of NingXia. Stress Away, Valor as needed and Sacred Mountain (one of my favorite oils!) in the diffuser.

Evening: I take Life 5 and put Cedarwood and Frankincense in the tub, Oregano on feet and JuvaFlex over lungs. Skincare regimen: Orange Blossom facial wash, ART Toner, homemade facial serum, Sheerlumé, Boswellia cream and Wolfberry eye cream.

What does Young Living mean to you? Young Living has been such an important part of the journey of discovery we are on as we really began to take ownership of our health and choices and ask important questions. Since I quit teaching and embarked on the homeschooling journey, the opportunities to involve our children and have both of us home with them has been amazing (and challenging at times, but leading to tremendous growth in character, patience and discipline: the one we are really focusing on currently). We are still working on finding balance and properly prioritizing our convictions and values. We love how Young Living fits within this lifestyle and worldview.

Chelsea Tudor
Platinum, Missouri

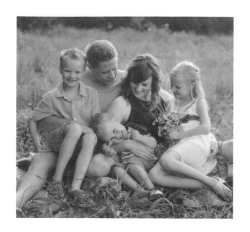

Young Living member since? 2013
Spouse: Dustin Tudor
Age: 31
Hobbies: Church, family, photography, camping, traveling
Favorite Young Living product?
Stress Away and NingXia Red
Favorite Young Living farm or event?
St Marie's Idaho Farm

Describe your day using Young Living products:

Morning: In the morning, I shower using Lavender shampoo and bath gel and apply Lavender lotion. I apply Frankincense and jojoba oil and ART Renewal Serum to my face and brush my teeth with Thieves AromaBright toothpaste. I drink one ounce of NingXia Red and take a Super C tablet. I apply Stress Away to my wrists and diffuser necklace and we diffuse an oil combination for the day!

Afternoon: We use Thieves cleaner for anything and everything because with 3 kiddos, something is always getting spilled, dirty or grimy! We love the smell and the fact that it is toxin free! We also use the Thieves dish soap and laundry detergent and love them both! I am constantly grabbing for whatever oils I feel like I need at the time both for myself and for my kids. My favorite mid-day snack is a Chocolate Coated Slique Bar! I am totally obsessed with them!

Evening: My kids use the entire KidScents line, including the oils and all of the bath and body products. They use they kids Slique toothpaste and we apply oils to all of our feet at bedtime every night. We always diffuse Lavender and Thieves at night for the kids and we usually diffuse Stress Away and Valor in our bedroom. I apply Progessence Plus right before bed and take a Life 5 capsule.

What does Young Living mean to you? Young Living has been life changing for our family in so many ways! First and foremost, it has allowed us to overhaul almost every area of our home to remove toxins. Young Living opened our eyes to the idea of truly having a chemical free home and a toxin free lifestyle. Young Living has helped us see that we are capable of replacing toxins in our home and life with products that are beneficial to us and I am so grateful! I know our family is better off for it!

Christa Smith

Royal Crown Diamond, Oklahoma

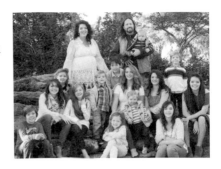

YL member since? 2009

Spouse: Jason Smith

Age: 897 in Parent Years (15 children)

Hobbies: Making children... you know it's a super power! Reading, singing, family dance offs, getting exercise in (I just started now that the baby is 4 months).

Favorite Young Living product? Peace & Calming, Peppermint

Favorite Young Living farm or event? Oh man, all of them... anytime you can get close to anyone from Young Living, but Convention & Beauty School. Getting to meet Gary and Mary for the first time was such an honor!

Describe your day using Young Living products:

Morning: I start the day with a NingXia Red, but each day is a little different. I believe in rotating and hitting your system with diversity. Thyromin, EndoGize. FemiGen or PD 80/20 depending on the needs of my system. Sometimes SclarEssence in my mouth too. BLM and Sulfurzyme! Essentialzyme to help with absorption. I pray Ephesians 6:13 while I use White Angelica. Wolfberry bar or ComforTone.

Afternoon. More maintenance or when I can get it them in... Lemon or Slique oil water. Slique tea all day. Three of my fave: Juvaflex, Brain Power and Clarity. NingXia Red package (and I have to hide them or they will bgone in one morning by our kids).

Evening: SleepEssence, Thyromin, AlkaLime and K & B if during cycle. A bath is my favorite wind down time... Lavender shampoo and conditioner. (The cool thing is that my hair, which used to be an everyday wash because of greasiness now only requires washing every 3-4 days). ART wash or Satin Mint scrub, followed with ART Serum or 3 Wise Men oil. (I love to rotate). I LOVE KidScents lotion or Cel-Lite Massage oil.

What does Young Living mean to you? Young Living is constantly thinking and caring about you. Through incentive trips, awards, conventions, trainings, farms, payout structure, it is clear they care a ton about you. You are the real product; the oils are just a side blessing. Never in any place in the world would I have an opportunity like Young Living has given me and my family! A stay at home mom of 15 now travels the world helping others. Young Living is unique; there is no competition.

Christi Collins
Diamond, Massachusetts

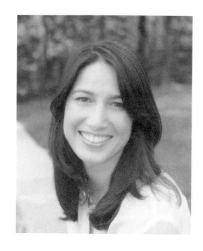

Young Living member since? 2007

Spouse: Ben Collins

Age: 39

Hobbies: Adventures with my boys, dates with husband, reading, a trained clairvoyant, Barre class. I love decluttering my home!

Favorite Young Living product?
Peppermint and ART Renewal Serum

Favorite Young Living product gift?
Thieves Household Cleaner

Favorite Young Living farm or event? The Ecuador Farm is out of this world!

Describe your day using Young Living products:

Morning Thieves bar soap, Peppermint/Lavender or Copaiba Vanilla shampoo and conditioner. Then Genesis lotion. For my face: ART Gentle Foaming Cleanser, Satin facial scrub (every other morning), ART Toner, Renewal Serum (I LOVE THIS!) ART moisturizer, and Wolfberry eye cream. Progessence Plus and then Endoflex over my throat. AromaBright toothpaste in the morning. DIY deodorant with AromaBright toothpaste, Petitgrain, Purification, & Lavender! I put AlkaLime in my first glass of water with a drop of Lemon. I take CortiStop, Super C and Essentialzyme, along with 2 NingXia Red. I take OmegaGize and before I start making breakfast and put oils in my Aria diffuser in my kitchen. As I work I like to diffuse Highest Potential, Magnify Your Purpose, Gathering or Clarity.

Evening: Life 5. For my face: ART Gentle Foaming Cleanser, Toner, Moisturizer with Frankincense, Boswellia Wrinkle Cream, and Wolfberry Eye Cream. I put Rose Ointment on my lips because it moisturizes all night long. I will apply Progessence Plus again. I put Cedarwood on the back of my neck, Lavender on my chest, and Valor or Peace & Calming on my wrists. If I really want to chill out before bed, I will put a drop of Vetiver on both big toes.

What does Young Living mean to you? Young Living means choices, time freedom, *major* personal growth, and an awesome community! Young Living has allowed me to take my passion for healthy living, make it a purposeful business, and in the process... change my life and the lives of others!

Claudia Dosamantes-Smeltzer

Diamond, Texas

Young Living member since? 2012

Spouse: Roger Smeltzer, Jr.

Age: 31

Hobbies: Reading and worship time with the kids. So fun to dance and worship with them.

Favorite Young Living product?

Nitro and NingXia Red

Favorite Young Living product gift?

Lavender

Favorite Young Living farm or event? Mona

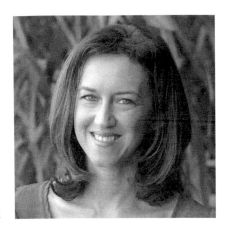

Describe your day using Young Living products:

Morning: Wake up and take Lemon in my water. Then a shot of NingXia Red with Nitro and Orange oil in water. Apply Clarity and Focus before I start the day. Diffuse in the kitchen with different. Take Young Living enzymes and brush with Thieves AromaBright toothpaste. We use all the household and bath Thieves line. Then usually Thieves, Valor, Lavender, Lemon and Peppermint or Vetiver with Cedarwood. Mid-morning snack includes a shot of NingXia Red with MindWise, Lemon and Peppermint. Also more Stress Away for mommy.

Afternoon: Lunch time includes another round of enzymes for all of us. Mom gets a dose of OmegaGize and so do the kids. I take a drop of Ocotea mid-afternoon to help maintain healthy blood sugar levels.

Evening: We take Young Living enzymes for dinner time. I use the ART cleanser and Boswellia wrinkle cream after shower. Bedtime oils for kids vary but include oils needed for support like RC, Thieves, Eucalyptus, etc. Mommy uses Thyromin at bedtime and Tranquil, Frankincense or Peace & Calming. Aroma Life over my heart and Cypress on my legs. We like to diffuse Lavender and Thieves for us at nighttime.

What does Young Living mean to you? Young Living is a way of life for us; a lifestyle! A lifestyle that has blessed us beyond what we could have imagined. It is a way of life that impacts more than just our health. It has had a great impact on our marriage, our relationships, friendships, time freedom, financial freedom, personal growth and our children's future! One simple choice, the choice to join Young Living and share our story, has moved mountains in our lives.

Corie DeVries
Diamond, Alaska

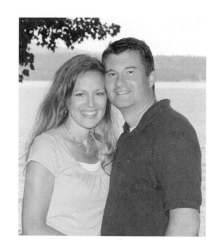

YL member since? 2009
Spouse: Gordon DeVries
Age: 37
Hobbies: Hiking, fishing, camping, bike riding, reading, writing
Favorite Young Living product? Valor
Favorite Product to Gift? Stress Away Roll On
Favorite Young Living farm or event? I love the quiet and solitude of the St. Maries farm.

Describe your day using Young Living products:

Morning: My routine often changes from day to day, but I use oils from sun up to sun down. I take water with Lemon, Life 5, Sulfurzyme, JuvaTone and enzymes. Valor, Sheerlumé on my face. I use Joy or Gentle Baby under my arms. Often we eat Einkorn pancakes and everyone takes their supplements at breakfast. MightyVites and Super C Chewable. I HAVE to have Super B, Mineral Essence, Longevity, Super C and NingXia. *Afternoon:* Time for another Nitro! This is when I reach for a "wake me up" oil, such as Peppermint or Motivation. I also love to apply Abundance. By this time, I am usually in need of my Deep Relief roll on or PanAway! My children often ask for Protein or Balance Complete for a snack. On warm days, they know to pull a NingXia Red packet out of the freezer and enjoy a healthy popsicle! We use the Thieves line for everything. *Evening:* Bath time means KidScents shampoo and the rest of us love our Lavender Volume shampoo and conditioner. My favorite soap right now is Sacred Mountain. Everyone oils up before bed! Thieves, Lavender, SleepyIze, and Tranquil roll on. Progessence Plus for Mama and Shutran for Daddy and then supplements again.

What does Young Living mean to you? Young Living means FREEDOM: freedom of time, freedom of health choices, freedom in choosing which activities and opportunities will best suit the needs of our family. Young Living's focus on Wellness, Purpose and Abundance in ALL areas of our lives has blessed our family in priceless, countless ways, and it is an absolute privilege, joy and BLESSING to be able to share that same opportunity with everyone around us!

Courtney Critz
Crown Diamond, Texas

Young Living member since? 2012

Spouse: John Critz

Age: 35

Hobbies: Travel, reading, house projects. This business has become my main hobby!

Favorite Young Living product? NingXia Red

Favorite Young Living farm or event? I loved being at the Mona Farm in the Utah mountains and attending my first convention last year.

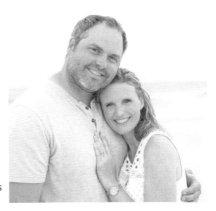

Describe your day using Young Living products:

Morning: Post workout drink with Balance Complete, Grapefruit oil, BLM (3 days a week), Young Living shampoo and conditioner, body wash, and Mint facial scrub, ART toner and moisturizer, Wolfberry eye cream. Mountain Mint deodorant, Sensation lotion, Progessence Plus, OolaFun (that's my current "F" needing the most balance). Thieves toothpaste and mouthwash, NingXia Red, Nitro if needed, and MindWise. We give our kids the above plus Life 5, BLM, MightyVites and MightyZyme. Everyone gets citrus oils in water. Hubs uses Shutran daily.

Afternoon: Throughout the day we use oils as needed, including Valor, Lavender, Motivation, Stress Away, Deep Relief, Balsam Fir and many others. Nitro when tired. Slique bars and Wolfberry Crisps often for snacks. Slique gum when craving something sweet. Something in diffuser like Sacred Mountain or Ylang Ylang. Thieves cleaner in my laundry loads and cleaning. Thieves hand sanitizer, mints and spray in my car for all errands.

Evening: Kids all have varying nightly oil routines based on current health and Zyto scan. SleepyIze, Tranquil, Thieves, Peace & Calming and more are commonly used. We often have the diffusers running in the bedrooms with calming oils.

What does Young Living mean to you? Freedom. To bless others, to be with my family, to pursue dreams of elaborate giving, loving, playing and traveling. Opportunity to build a business with my husband and my kids and a lifestyle of wellness, purpose and abundance that equips us for anywhere God sends us!

Cristy Jenkins
Platinum, Alabama

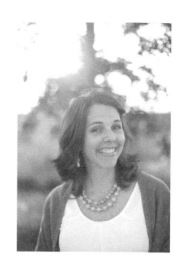

Young Living member since? 2013
Spouse: Andrew Jenkins
Age: 39
Children: 9 (Ages 2 to 14)
Hobbies: Doula, childbirth education, hiking and frisbee golf with my family, trips with Andrew, beach with my family.
Favorite Young Living product? Nitro, DiGize, Lavender, NingXia Red or Power Meal

Favorite Young Living farm or event?
Event: Drive to Win in Hawaii. Farm: Ecuador

Describe your day using Young Living products:
Morning: Morning Start Bath & Shower Gel, Lavender lotion, Orange Blossom face wash, ART Toner, ART moisturizers (in summer), Sheerlumé, Sandalwood Moisture cream (winter), PD 80/20, Master Formula, EndoGize, Sulfurzyme, MultiGreens, Nitro. En-R-Gee, OolaFitness on feet before workout and Power Meal with NingXia Red after.
Afternoon: MultiGreens, Sulfurzyme, Master Formula, Longevity, Super B, Nitro
Evening: Super Cal, Thyromin, Mineral Essence, Rehemogen, NingXia Red, Life 5, Orange Blossom face wash, ART Toner, ART or Sandalwood moisturizer.
When Traveling: I have a morning/lunch/evening "pill" case for all my supplements. Plus, I add DiGize and Thieves spray, lozenges and hand purifier. Also: Thieves, Peace & Calming, Valor, Roman Chamomile, Peppermint, Lavender, Lemon and RC.
What does Young Living mean to you? Young Living means health and wellness for me and my family! It means walking in wholeness and being confident in our healthcare. In addition, it means FREEDOM and simplicity. We have been blessed with new friendships, new products to help support our bodies and a financial freedom we've never experienced. Young Living means integrity, honor and diligence. It means building bridges towards the skeptics, fearful and apprehensive all around us; it is freedom and walking in it with humble confidence extending grace along the journey.
What is your favorite clean eating meal? Create-your-own salad with the family!!

Crystal Burchfield

Crown Diamond, Missouri

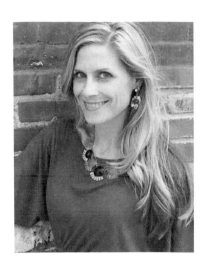

Young Living member since? 2011

Spouse: Verick Burchfield

Age: 37

Kids: 4 (ages 5 to 15)

Hobbies: Being outside, going on walks, reading and writing in the evening energizes me.

Favorite Young Living product? NingXia Red

Favorite Young Living product to gift?
Orb diffuser with a bottle of oil

Favorite Young Living farm or event?
Provence, France farm

Describe your day using Young Living products:

Morning: I love to start my day off with a Power Meal shake! I typically apply oils like Joy, Highest Potential and Abundance in the mornings, Thieves household products.

Afternoon: I love NingXia Red around 2 or 3 pm. Sometimes I take it in the morning AND afternoon! I may add a drop of Orange or Tangerine oil to it.

Evening: Depending on my mood, I may use oils like Peppermint to help promote late night wakefulness when I'm working, or Valor and RutaVaLa to help me relax when turning in for the night. I love ImmuPro and SleepEssence, the ART Masque, Sheerlumé (which I LOVE) and other oils on my face! Also, I love Valor soap and Lavender lotion.

When Traveling: I usually take two pouches of NingXia a day when traveling, a Nitro tube if I have to stay up later than usual, and I NEVER leave home without DiGize! Lavender and Thieves and of course my Thieves sanitizer are must haves. I love oils that have calming scents like Tranquil and Stress Away. At night before bed, it helps to have SleepEssence to promote a good night's rest in a new environment.

What does Young Living mean to you? Before Young Living, my family was trying to walk a path of wellness haphazardly that we had no GPS for. We are so thankful to have found a company that helps us accomplish many of our goals all in one! Less toxins: check. Optimizing wellness with supplements and products: check. OOLA Life balance: check. Fellowship with like-minded families on the same journey: check. A message of giving back and caring for others all over the world: check. Young Living is a lifestyle that you want to live and share!

What is your favorite clean eating meal? I LOVE a good salad!

Danette Goodyear
Crown Diamond, Texas

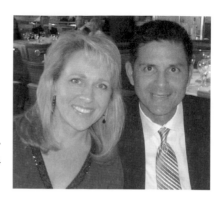

Young Living member since? 2003
Spouse: Jim Goodyear
Age: 48
Hobbies: Travel, tennis, watercolor painting, being outdoors, hiking, and antique hunting.
Favorite Young Living product?
MultiGreens and ImmuPower
Favorite Young Living farm or event? France and Ecuador Farms

Describe your day using Young Living products:

Morning: Lemon oil in water, NingXia Red, MindWise, Rehemogen, Mineral Essence. Sulfurzyme, BLM, MultiGreens. Essentialzymes-4, OmegaGize, SuperCal, Super C. Often, Einkorn pancakes with Agave nectar. AromaBright toothpaste and Thieves mouthwash. Sensation body wash, Copaiba Vanilla shampoo and conditioner, Orange Blossom face wash. Lavender lip balm. Dentarome Plus toothpaste under arms (as deodorant). Frankincense, Geranium and Lavender oils on face. ART Renewal Serum. Sheerlumé under eyes. Endoflex over thyroid and adrenals. Valor on feet. White Angelica on shoulders and over heart. Abundance (from feet to head), Humility and Inspiration, Motivation, or Envision. Lavender lotion. And as perfume: One Gift, Highest Potential or Stress Away.

Afternoon: I'll brush my teeth with AromaBright. Enjoy some NingXia, a Slique bar or Wolfberry bar. Diffuse: Clarity, Thieves, Abundance, Purification. Thieves spray, purifier and household products all throughout the day.

Evening: AromaBright toothpaste and Thieves mouthwash. Wash face with Thieves hand soap or ART Gentle Cleanser. Young Living lip balm. Wolfberry eye cream, Frankincense, Lavender and Progessence on skin. ImmuPower and Valor on feet, Idaho Blue Spruce on ankles. Endoflex again. Cedarwood on forehead. JuvaTone tabs, Life 5, SuperCal and as needed, CortiStop or Thyromin. Middle of night: Essentialzyme or Detoxzyme (I alternate).

What does Young Living mean to you? Young Living has meant a huge improvement in my health, in my personal growth and in my family's abundance. Jim and I both retired from our previous jobs. We are forever grateful!

Debbie Erickson
Diamond, Texas

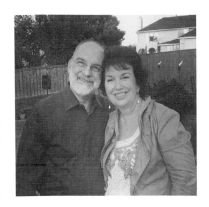

Young Living member since? 2011

Spouse: Daniel Erickson

Hobbies: Having fun with our family and great friends, swimming, walking, traveling all over the world, teaching and presenting on natural health topics, ministry, our black labs, a good movie, a good book, many different music genres; we love our church!

Favorite Young Living product? NingXia Red

Favorite Young Living farm or event? Farms in Utah and Idaho, and every Convention.

Describe your day using Young Living products:

Morning: Water with a few drops of citrus oil. NingXia Red and healthy foods (the Einkorn Pancake & Waffle Mix is absolutely delicious!). Master Formula, Life 5, OmegaGize, and we use Essentialzymes-4 and MindWise. Peppermint and DiGize essential oils after each meal. Boswellia Wrinkle Cream. AromaBright toothpaste. We have oils and at least one diffuser in each room and frequently have multiple diffusers going.

Afternoon: Slique bars are the best meal replacement ever! They taste great and really satisfy. I also love to sip on Slique tea, hot or iced. I take a NingXia Nitro and another 2 ounces of NingXia Red for a pick-me-up. For concentration, I sip citrus oils in water and diffuse oils next to my computer in my office. Essential oils in water are great for hydration, concentration, energy, focus and appetite control. Thieves Household Cleaner has helped us eliminate all other types of cleaning products and we love that!

Evening: At bedtime, I take several Sulfurzyme and BLM capsules, Master Formula, and Longevity. I often diffuse next to our bed. I also use AromaBright toothpaste, Wolfberry Eye Cream, and essential oils on the soles of my feet. I love Aroma Life, Stress Away, Peace & Calming, Valor, and Frankincense for a restful sleep.

What does Young Living mean to you? Young Living means, to me, many of our dreams coming true! I am an RN, but I get to help even more people achieve wellness doing what I do in Young Living than I ever did as a nurse! I love sharing natural health with people! I love empowering people to help them make wise health choices. I love working with our amazing Young Living team!

Debra Raybern

Royal Crown Diamond, Texas

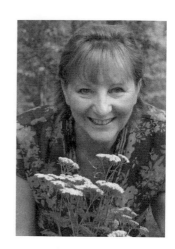

Young Living member since? 2000
Hobbies: Sewing, quilting, crochet, reading
Favorite Young Living product?
ImmuPower blend
Favorite Young Living farm or event?
Convention

Describe your day using Young Living products:

Morning: AromaBright toothpaste, Thieves mouthwash and floss, Abundance (wrists), White Angelica (head/shoulders), and Valor (back of neck). Motivation, Into the Future, ImmuPower and Sacred Mountain. Wash face with Orange Blossom, Young Living toner, and Boswellia for moisturizer. Lavender or Genesis lotion are my body lotions. Mountain Mist and/or LavaDerm Mist over the face. Add Lemon, Ocotea and/or JuvaCleanse to water, NingXia Red, or in a capsule. Hands are always washed with Thieves Foaming Hand Soap, Thieves home products for the house.

Afternoon: Longevity, Inner Defense, BLM, Essentialzyme and Master Formula at lunch. Stress Away, Inspiration and Oola Field. Before exercise Oola Fitness. After exercise Balance Complete, PowerMeal, protein shake or a Wolfberry snack bar. Shower using Morning Start, the Copaiba hair products, more body lotion and redo the facial moisturizer. I have my own muscle blend for knees, shoulders, etc. (depending on the workout) and apply this blend topically and top with a few drops Ortho Sport.

Evening: Sulfurzyme, Life 5, OmegaGize, ComforTone, BLM, Super Cal, Master Formula and whatever else I think is needed.

What does Young Living mean to you? Young Living means I can enjoy great natural wellness products, allowing me to live life to the fullest. I also get to share them with others and have the financial abundance for my family, and am able to liberally donate to my church, ministries and organizations near to my heart. Young Living has allowed me the pleasure of growing as a person, business woman, friend and mom. Through Young Living, I have friends all around the world, which I would never have had otherwise. Young Living is a blessing!

Erica Mallon

Silver, New Jersey

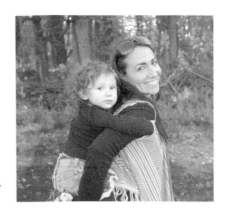

Young Living member since? 2014

Spouse: Randy Mallon

Age: 33

Hobbies: DIY projects, camping, crafting, dance and family time!

Favorite Young Living product? Stress Away, Inner Defense, NingXia Nitro & ALL THINGS Thieves!!!

Favorite YL product to gift someone? NingXia Nitro, Stress Away, Breathe Again and Deep Relief,

Describe your day using Young Living products:

Morning: I start my day with Thieves toothpaste and the ART line. I use homemade deodorant, hair detangler spray, pest-repellent and sun lotion that I made with a few simple ingredients and Young Living essential oils. I apply Stress Away (wrists), Valor (back of neck), citrus oils (behind our ears/sides of neck). I diffuse Citrus Fresh, Believe, or Lavender! I'll use RepelAroma for our Bulldog. NingXia Red and a capsule of Copaiba, Lemon and Peppermint. Super C chewable, OmegaGize and MultiGreens. Sometimes an Inner Defense capsule. Water with Lemon oil.

Afternoon: Re-apply oils and take a NingXia Nitro. I diffuse Thieves in our living room, if we have visitors or a playdate (to boost immune system), and I clean up the kitchen, bathrooms & toy room with Thieves cleaner!

Evening: Diffuse Stress Away after husband's 3-hour commute. I often cook or bake with essential oils. Husband: Mister oil and Life 5 probiotic before bed. Toddler: bath with Lavender or Peace & Calming. I will put the diffuser in the bedrooms with Thieves. We apply Valor, PanAway, or Aroma Siez for tired muscles. Thieves, Oregano, Lemongrass for immune support.

What does Young Living mean to you? Young Living is a way of life. It has literally changed the way we live our daily lives as individuals and as a family. We have been able to slowly, but progressively rid our home of toxins and replace them with safe, natural products from a company who cares about integrity as well as the health and safety of its customers. Young Living is a lifestyle!

Erin Rodgers
Diamond, Tennessee

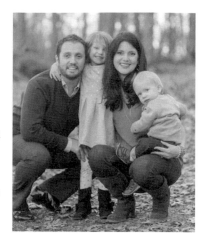

Young Living member since? 2014
Spouse: Bronce Rodgers
Age: 35
Hobbies: Reading, photography, traveling with my family
Favorite Young Living product?
Thieves, Lavender, Longevity and MultiGreens
Favorite Young Living farm or event?
Favorite event was the Global Leadership Cruise 2015
Describe your day using Young Living products:

Morning: NingXia Red all day, every day. Thieves, Joy or a citrus oil in the diffuser, Happy blend on my kids (Stress Away, Valor, Lavender in a roller, diluted), White Angelica on my wrists and jaw line to relax and calm down for the day. Supplements: Longevity, MultiGreens, True Source, OmegaGize. I wash the counters with Thieves Cleaner. Sheerlumé on my face. We have Thieves Hand Soap at every sink.

Afternoon: Catch up on my supplements if I forgot them in the morning! En-R-Gee under my big toe to get stuff done. We use Thieves Spray and hand purifier in the car, I keep some in the car and in my purse. Lavender oil roller and KidScents oils roller stay in my purse too and are used regularly. Diffuse something in the kitchen… varies everyday based on my mood.

Evening: Tons of shower products such as Lavender Mint shampoo and conditioner, Satin Mint facial scrub, ART system and Sheerlumé, occasional ART Creme Masque. Diffusers in kids' rooms with Thieves and Lavender. Diffuser in our room: Peace & Calming and Lavender.

What does Young Living mean to you? We always strived to be "healthy" and "natural" but the world of Young Living essential oils has opened up a whole new approach to wellness. Combined with the business side, we are experiencing the Lord's blessing on us all, "beyond what we asked for or imagined" (Ephesians 3:20). We are so grateful!

Ernie Yarbrough

Crown Diamond, Alabama

YL member since? August 2012
Spouse: Myra Yarbrough
Age: 33
Hobbies: Reading, CrossFit, running and computer coding
Favorite Young Living product? Thieves
Favorite Young Living farm or event?
Highland Flats Farm

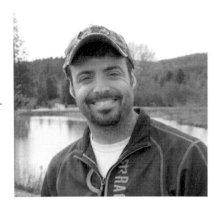

Describe your day using Young Living products:

Morning: I drink NingXia Red with a varying combination of Orange, Lime and Cinnamon Bark. We run several diffusers, but I especially enjoy running the Rainstone diffuser in my office with Magnify Your Purpose. I also take BLM, Master Formula, Super C and Sulfurzyme.

Afternoon: I apply Valor, Shutran and Idaho Blue Spruce regularly throughout the afternoon as needed. I also take Lemon in my water.

Evening: I often enjoy a Pure Protein Complete for an evening meal replacement. I brush with Thieves Dentarome and use Young Living dental floss as well as applying oils to my feet. I enjoy using Lavender, Cedarwood or Peace & Calming in the bedroom diffuser.

What does Young Living mean to you? Young Living has been a perfect fit for us because it supplied the healthy options we needed that fit into our active lifestyle as a family. Young Living has blessed our family by allowing us to care for all the normal needs of health and wellness in a natural and effective way while also bringing me home from my previous job to work the Young Living business with my wife and pursue our life dreams together with our growing family.

What is your favorite clean eating meal? Breakfast. I love eating farm fresh eggs, organic bacon, vegetables, and fruit. Occasionally we will mix it up with Einkorn wheat pancakes or waffles and Gary's NingXia Berry Syrup!

Evangeline Reed

Diamond, Texas

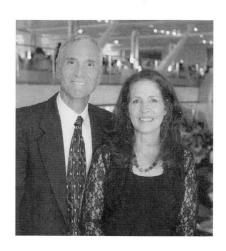

Young Living member since? 2006
Spouse: Dr. Thomas Reed
Age: 54
Hobbies: Reading, organic cooking and baking, farming, sustainable living
Favorite Young Living product?
Christmas Spirit
Favorite Young Living farm or event?
We fulfilled a lifelong dream to visit France when we visited the farm in France this year.

Describe your day using Young Living products:

Morning: First: Nitro and NingXia. Tbsp of ICP in apple juice. Dentarome Ultra, Thieves Mouthwash, and any Young Living shower gel along with one of the shampoos and conditioners. Then 10 drops of citrus oils with Cel-Lite Magic. ART toner and skin oils (Sandalwood, Frankincense, Bergamot, Cistus and others) followed by ART Renewal Serum, Moisturizer and Eye Cream. Lavender Lip Balm. A small dab of the Dentarome Plus mixed with water for an underarm deodorant. Joy, Hope, Magnify Your Purpose, Valor and Abundance oils. Sometimes Einkorn Pancake Mix and Wolfberry Syrup. Sulfurzyme, BLM, Essentialzyme, OmegaGize, Super B and C, Master Formula, EndoGize, MultiGreens, Longevity. Young Living shake.

Afternoon: I get my diffuser going with Clarity, Slique and Christmas Spirit. I use BLM, NingXia Red and Nitro. NingXia and Nitro in my car and in my purse so that if I am out and about I have some. I carry oils and Lavender lotion with me everywhere. We use Thieves cleaner, spray, hand soap, sanitizer, etc. throughout the day.

Evening: BLM, Life 5. ART Foaming Cleanser and moisturizer then Frankincense, Sandalwood, Cistus and Bergamot. Thyme and Valor to my feet and diffuse Peace & Calming or Lavender or take a SleepEssence. I take about 10-12 Detoxzyme before bed along with Thyromin. Sometimes Epsom salt baths and a favorite oil or two.

What does Young Living mean to you? Not only have Young Living products improved our health, but learning to share them with others has grown me as a person and allowed my husband and I to experience things that we have only dreamed of. Young Living has become a vehicle for allowing us bless others in very tangible ways—which is such a joy. What fun seeing those dreams come true!

Gregg Johnson

Royal Crown Diamond, Colorado

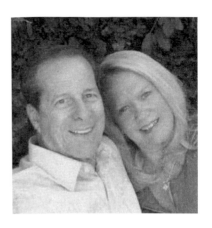

Young Living member since? 1996

Spouse: Carol Johnson

Age: 64

Hobbies: Golf and family. Travel between two homes in Colorado and Arizona.

Favorite Young Living product?
NingXia Red, St. Maries Lavender, Valor

Favorite Product to Gift? St. Maries Lavender

Favorite Young Living farm or event? Highland Flats Winter Harvest

Describe your day using Young Living products:

Morning: Young Living Lavender shower gel, Young Living Copaiba Vanilla shampoo and NingXia Red.

Afternoon: Whatever oils strike me at the time. It varies each day. Essentialzyme for sure after every meal!

Evening: NingXia Red, Essentialzyme, Valor, Lavender, Life 5 after dinner.

When Traveling: All the same daily routine but when we are staying in hotels, we use the diffuser with purification oil to purify any musty smells.

What does Young Living mean to you? For us, Young Living means allowing us to have the ability to help people change their lives and the lives of others and help them find success.

What is your favorite clean eating meal? We love all kinds of fish and we also love a nice chicken Caesar salad.

Hailey Aliff
Diamond, Louisiana

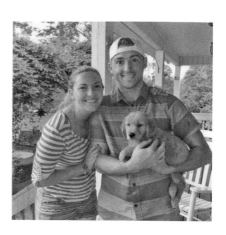

Young Living member since? 2013
Spouse: Jeremy Aliff
Age: 26
Hobbies: Volleyball, midwife assistant/doula, outdoor adventures like hiking and camping
Favorite Young Living product? NingXia Red with lots of oils added to it
Favorite YL product to gift someone? Deep Relief roll on

Favorite Young Living farm or event? The Ecuador Farm and the Melissa Harvest at the St. Maries, Idaho farm is my favorite event.

Describe your day using Young Living products:

Morning: NingXia Red with Orange oil or Thieves or Peppermint. I rub Joy on my heart and En-R-Gee on my wrists. I usually drop one oil drop on my diffuser necklace and take Master Formula daily. A favorite lately is "Build Your Dream" or "Valor II". My husband uses Shutran or Idaho Blue Spruce and is currently taking the Life 5 probiotic daily.

Afternoon: We both drink oily water throughout the day with citrus oils. When I work from home, I diffuse Lavender or Ylang Ylang and Lemon Myrtle around the clock. We take NingXia Nitro for a boost.

Evening: We take NingXia with Lavender or Chamomile in it. I put oils on my feet and Tranquil roll on around my neck and back of my ears. Jeremy rubs on Vetiver and Cedarwood. We have lots of oil-concoctions in roller balls that we made each for a different purpose. A favorite nighttime diffusing combo is Patchouli + Lavender or even Peace & Calming II.

What does Young Living mean to you? Young Living means purity and integrity. It gives hope to so many people—physically, emotionally and financially. It means purpose and wellness and abundance, just like their tagline says. Our family is forever changed thanks to Young Living.

What is your favorite clean eating meal? I just love a good salad.

Heather Brock
Diamond, California

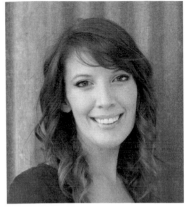

Young Living member since? 2012

Spouse: John Brock

Age: 37

Hobbies: Children, homeschooling, church activities, healthy restaurants, live music and musicals, raising chickens and playing board games or chess.

Favorite Young Living product? The Aria Premium Starter Kit

Favorite YL product to gift someone? A diffuser or NingXia

Favorite Young Living farm or event? Convention!

Describe your day using Young Living products:

Morning: Diffuse oil. Brush with Thieves AromaBright. Shower and/or washing with Lavender shampoo and conditioner, one of the luxurious body washes and Orange Blossom facial wash. I use Thieves toothpaste as deodorant and put Sheerlumé and a touch of Frankincense on my face. I take Super B, NingXia Red, and Essentialzyme and/or Sulfurzyme with food. I will oil up our children as needed. A little Clarity for spelling lessons, Harmony or Joy to help sibling relationships, Brain Power for Math. TummyGize or Peppermint after breakfast. We put Thieves in the chicken's water.

Afternoon: NingXia Nitro, NingXia Red and any one of these: BLM, OmegaGize, MultiGreens, Mega Cal, Super C. Diffuse oil in a different part of the house according to the needs of the family. After lunch: a little Peppermint, DiGize or TummyGize.

Evening: A warm cup of tea with a favorite oil in it. Sometimes we even skip the tea and just drink a warm cup of water with oil. I will oil up my kids to encourage restful sleep and healthy immune systems. A little Progessence Plus for me, Shutran for him. Evening supplements may include Life 5, Longevity, ImmuPro and another shot of NingXia!

What does Young Living mean to you? Wellness, Purpose and Abundance! Honestly, when I started I did not get that slogan at all! Not only did Young Living change the environment of our home, it supports us in mind, body and spirit like nothing else! Young Living gave us a new perspective on serving and helping people, and on true abundance and freedom.

Heather Doll
Diamond, Canada

Young Living member since? 2013
Spouse: Wade Doll
Age: 46
Hobbies: Traveling in our motorhome, reading, curling, golfing, spending lots of time with friends and family.
Favorite Young Living product? ImmuPro
Favorite YL product to gift someone? Thieves Household Cleaner
Favorite Young Living farm or event? Diamond trip to Paris

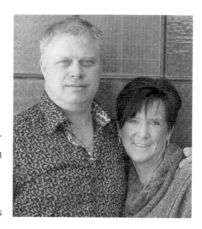

Describe your day using Young Living products:

Morning: Shower with Young Living shampoo and conditioner and bath gel. Drink NingXia, take supplements (OmegaGize, Sulfurzyme, BLM, SuperCal, MultiGreens, Super B & Super C). Sometimes I will take a capful of Lemon, Peppermint and use Lavender. Every day I make up a water bottle with Grapefruit, Orange and Lemon in it.
Afternoon: Drink NingXia Red and Nitro, make another water bottle up with Grapefruit, Orange and Lemon in it.
Evening: In the evening I take Detoxzyme and Life 5 and ImmuPro.

What does Young Living mean to you? Young Living has given my family and me a greater purpose in life. We love the freedom that Young Living allows us by traveling and sharing the amazing products. I do not consider this a job because I am having too much fun! We have made a lot of new friends and are enjoying a much healthier lifestyle. I am excited that our kids are growing up with Young Living in their life and love to share the products with friends and family, too. It is exciting to see them reach for a Young Living product first and not even consider the alternatives!

What is your favorite clean eating meal? My favorite clean eating meal is a glass of vegetable & fruit juice (that I juice in my juicer), a fresh garden salad (without dressing) and a big glass of water.

Heather Portwood
Diamond, Oklahoma

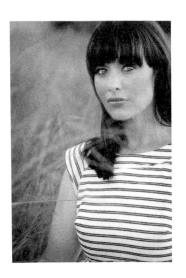

Young Living member since? 2011

Spouse: Christian Portwood

Age: 38

Hobbies: With kids: coloring, playdoh, going to the zoo. Alone: good coffee, shopping at local shops, anywhere outside by the water.

Favorite Young Living product?
Frankincense

Favorite YL product to gift someone? Emotional oils, Abundance and Awaken.

Favorite Young Living farm or event? Diamond Trip to Croatia and Paris

Describe your day using Young Living products.

Morning: I will put 3-4 drops of a citrus oil on my belly, Endoflex on neck, Gratitude over my heart and then take MultiGreens, Sulfurzyme, NingXia Red, FemiGen. Facial products: Orange Blossom face wash, Satin Mint scrub, Wolfberry eye cream and Sandalwood moisturizer. Cel-Lite Magic as my lotion. I use Thieves toothpaste and mouthwash.

Afternoon: Diffuse Gathering or Stress Away I'll take Super B, Enzymes, OmegaGize, Nitro and Lemon and Grapefruit in water. Apply Envision, Magnify Your Purpose or Abundance.

Evening: Life 5, Detoxzyme, Thyromin and ImmuPro. Diffuse Lavender, ImmuPower, Tranquil sometimes SleepEssence.

When Traveling: I take everything with me, and then some. My vacation looks about the same as my daily routine.

What does Young Living mean to you? I do give all the glory to God for all the ways Young Living has enriched my life. This company and its products came at a time in my life that was full of hopeless desperation. Young Living, to me, means freedom and hope.

What is your favorite clean eating meal? Chinese Chicken salad with Brussels sprouts. Seriously could eat it for every meal.

Heidi Ross
Diamond, Canada

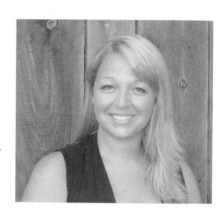

Young Living member since? 2012
Spouse: Rory Ross
Age: 34
Hobbies: Children, traveling, down-hill skiing, anything that pertains to health and wellness
Favorite Young Living product?
Highest Potential
Favorite Young Living farm or event? Hawaiian Sandalwood Farm

Describe your day using Young Living products:

Morning: Orange Blossom Face wash, toner, and ART light moisturizer with a drop of whatever oil I feel like that day. Every few days I add in the Satin Mint scrub. I love Thieves AromaBright toothpaste. My shampoo and conditioner, bath and shower gel, soaps and cleaners are all Young Living. Each day it might not be the same scent, but it's all Young Living. I also take NingXia Red, Super B & C, PD 80/20, Pure Protein with almond milk and some kind of fruit.

Afternoon: Super B, PD 80/20, Nitro, and more NingXia Red if I feel like it.

Evening: Life 5, ImmuPro and PD 80/20. (This all changes with the seasons, winter time a LOT more is added in!)

When Traveling: Life 5 and LOTS of it! Longevity or Inner Defense, and oils on the feet like ImmuPower. Diffusing is an ALL day event in our house. We have them in every room and sometimes more than one in a room! I LOVE our house smelling great!

What does Young Living mean to you? Young Living is a lifestyle. I grew up in a family where my parents had a small hobby farm. We raised most all our own food. So when I had my own family, a lot of those values have come back around and Young Living fits in with them! We use Young Living in everything because it's about the whole lifestyle. Taking out everything synthetic from our lifestyle and having healthy options is what this is about. Knowing I have a company that I can trust that has honesty and integrity behind it is why I chose Young Living.

What is your favorite clean eating meal? For breakfast, I'll have some kind of Young Living shake with fruit. Any other meal: Salad! I. LOVE. SALADS!

Jake Dempsey

Crown Diamond, Texas

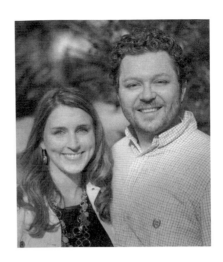

YL member since? April 2012

Spouse: Kristy Dempsey

Age: 34

Hobbies: I'm a nerd. Most of my time is spent writing software (like creating Oily Tools) or writing my book (an overview of the comp plan: www.imdrivenforsuccess.com) I also love anything related to cars. It's addicting.

Favorite Young Living product? NingXia

Describe your day using Young Living products:

Morning: Young Living shampoos, conditioners and body wash. My favorites are the Copaiba Vanilla Shampoo and Morning Start body wash and Orange Blossom face wash. (I also like the ART Gentle Cleanser—it's not just for girls!). Thieves Dentarome Ultra or AromaBright toothpaste. Then Idaho Blue Spruce and Shutran to my forearms and face as a cologne. Balance Complete shake every morning.

Afternoon: Each day I take BLM, MultiGreens, Inner Defense, Longevity, ComforTone, Sulfurzyme and Essentialzyme taken with 2-4 oz NingXia Red, Nitro & a citrus oil in water (my favorite drink)! I LOVE to diffuse Purification. We also have a Thieves foaming soap dispenser at every sink and clean only with the Thieves products!

Evening: More supplements along with another big bottle of NingXia water (without Nitro). If I had a big lunch I will also repeat my Balance Complete shake. Sometimes I'll have a treat like the Young Living Ecuadorian Dark Chocolessence.

When Traveling: We carry many of our Young Living products with us and always have a ton of oils with us. We probably use Thieves more than any other product while traveling: Hand Sanitizer, Mouth Spray, Lozenges, Mints.

What does Young Living mean to you? To me, Young Living is a lifestyle. Before Young Living, I was not as concerned about the effects of harsh chemicals on my family. Now I am grateful for Young Living's great products we can use to replace all those chemicals. I love that I can support my body and emotional health with oils and can use cleaning and personal care products and not worry about their effect on my or my children's bodies, or the environment.

What is your favorite clean eating meal? Right now, my favorite meal is my daily Balance Complete shake. A close second would be a salad at Snappy Salads.

James McDonald
Diamond, Illinois

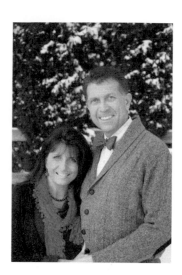

Young Living member since? 2010
Spouse: Stacy McDonald
Age: 55
Hobbies: Reading, traveling, power walking, hiking
Children: 10 (Ages 10 to 32)
Favorite Young Living product? Peppermint
Favorite Young Living farm or event?
St. Maries, Idaho farm and Drive to Win event in Hawaii

Describe your day using Young Living products:

Morning: Before my run, I use Balance Complete or Power Meal, NingXia Red and RC. After my shower, I take the following supplements: Master Formula, OmegaGize, BLM and Super B. I typically use Shutran, Sacred Frankincense and Tea Tree.

Afternoon: Throughout the day, I drink about a gallon of water. Often, I will put two drops of Peppermint into a 20 ounce bottle to support my alertness. I'll also occasionally reach for a NingXia Nitro. Mid-afternoon, I'm often grabbing a Wolfberry Crisp bar.

Evening: Essentialzyme after meals. Valor, Three Wise Men, or Sandalwood before bed.

What does Young Living mean to you? Wellness: With Young Living, I've seen improved wellness! I've dropped weight and seen renewed energy! Purpose: My life's goal has been to help others. Stacy and I do this now every day! Abundance: At one point, I thought I would never have the funds to retire. Now, I'm living as if retired, but helping many people! And as we do Young Living together, Stacy and I are closer than ever! This is real living with Young Living!

What is your favorite clean eating meal? Pretty much anything Stacy makes. She is an amazing cook and works hard to make sure we eat healthy meals. That being said, a smoked salmon salad can't be beat!

Jamie Flaman
Diamond, Canada

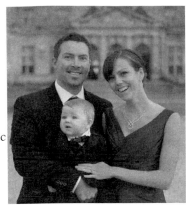

Young Living member since? 2012
Spouse: Chelsea Flaman
Age: 30
Hobbies: Family, baseball, football, graphic design, personal and leadership development
Favorite Young Living product?
NingXia Nitro and Deep Relief
Favorite Young Living product gift?
Peppermint
Favorite Young Living farm or event?
Ecuador

Describe your day using Young Living products:

Morning: AromaBright toothpaste, Thieves floss, Morning Start body wash, Pure Protein Complete with MindWise, Nitro and NingXia, MultiGreens, Super B, Super C and Sulfurzyme.

Afternoon: Oils are awesome in the diffuser, in the car, at work or at home. I lean towards diffusing a citrus oil to wake me up! I use Nitro in the afternoon if I'm dragging and need a kick!

Evening: Same supplements as in the morning: NingXia, Shutran and Deep Relief (for sore muscles).

When Traveling: Everyday oils kit or even Aroma Complete (never know when you need a specific oil!) Also carry Nitro and NingXia singles. Slique Bars, too!

What does Young Living mean to you? When I think of Young Living, I picture the farm and Gary and Mary leading the way on the tractor with the distributors in the field. I love this image, because it shows me how much care, attention and love goes into every product, and that the company is not seeking profit as much as they are seeking to make every single user of the product abundantly healthy and well! I think of great integrity and work ethic and I am very appreciative and grateful for all that Young Living has to offer! What an amazing company to journey with!

Janelle Chambers
Platinum, Missouri

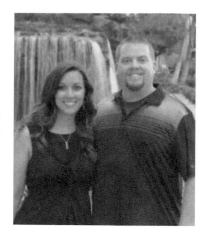

Young Living member since? June 2013

Spouse: Barry Chambers

Hobbies: We love card playing, bonfires, zip lining, games that challenge our minds, and just spending time with family & friends

Favorite Young Living product?
Nearly impossible to pick!

Favorite Young Living product to gift?
Peppermint and Lavender!

Favorite Young Living farm or event?
Ecuador Farm for sure!

Describe your day using Young Living products:

Morning: My daily use of oils & products change greatly depending on seasons of the year and what body systems need extra attention. Here are some of my tried & true favorites: All kit oils, Ylang Ylang, Stress Away, Myrrh, Orange, Oregano, Wintergreen, Awaken, Build Your Dream, Highest Potential, Humility, Joy, Motivation, Peace & Calming, Release, Valor, Deep Relief, Sleep Essence, Slique Tea, Balance Complete, Nitro, Ortho Ease Massage Oil, Rose Ointment. Purification & Frankincense in a DIY deodorant recipe, Sensation Bath & Shower Gel, Thieves Dentarome Ultra toothpaste, Lavender lotion, NingXia Red, V-6 oil as needed and ART Renewal Serum.

Afternoon: Breathe Again, White Angelica, Thieves Household Cleaner, Thieves Foaming Hand soap (throughout the day), True Source Vitamins, Vanilla Mint Lip Balm.

Evening: Frankincense, Thieves Dentarome Ultra Toothpaste, Orange Blossom Facial Wash, Sandalwood Moisture Cream

What does Young Living mean to you? Having Young Living in our lives means we no longer have to worry about the safety of products that our family uses for our health and wellness. It means we no longer have to suffer through things the way we used to because we wanted to avoid the only options we thought we had: toxic ones. It also means my family has financial peace and the ability to fulfill a dream we have to help further the Kingdom of God. It short, it means my life is forever changed in every way, and I am forever grateful!

What is your favorite clean eating meal? 2-ingredient pancakes is a favorite in our house! Bananas + eggs = delicious pancakes!

Jason Haymes
Platinum, Missouri

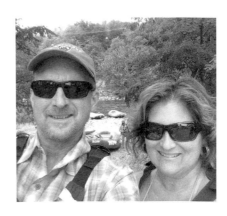

Young Living member since? 2013

Spouse: Krista Haymes

Age: 54

Children: Lindsay Haymes, Jordan Schrandt, Kate Haymes and Seth Haymes.

Hobbies: Working on our farm, shooting, running, flying airplanes, reading, traveling.

Favorite Young Living product?

Valor and NingXia

Describe your day using Young Living products:

Morning: I like to take En-R-Gee and NingXia Nitro before I run, then I shower with Valor bar soap and Lavender shampoo and conditioner. I use Thieves toothpaste and mouthwash and AromaGuard deodorant. I will drink one ounce of NingXia Red and take Master Formula, OmegaGize and Longevity supplements. I take and greatly value Lemongrass, Sage, Idaho Blue Spruce and a citrus oil in a capsule and topically apply Lavender, Frankincense, Shutran, Highest Potential and Helichrysum, then Ortho Ease on my knees as well as a few of my favorite oils. Peppermint is in my water all day.

Afternoon: Slique tea and Slique bars are a favorite. I apply oils topically as needed; usually Oola Balance, Valor and Peppermint.

Evening: Supplements: Master Formula, OmegaGize and Life 5. I apply Cedarwood topically and may use Frankincense topically or in the diffuser depending what I'm doing. Otherwise I diffuse any oil that will help us relax and unwind.

What does Young Living mean to you? I believe that God has been preparing me to talk about Young Living Essential Oils all my life. I became interested in medicinal plants when my grandfather took me up in the mountains of northern Arkansas gathering ginseng and goldenseal and sharing his knowledge of plants and their historic uses. I studied agriculture in college and have spent the last 27 years fostering a love for the land, plants and animals and encouraging young people's interest in agriculture. When I was introduced to Young Living, I didn't know what an essential oil was. But what I learned resonated with me and it felt like I had come full circle. From my grandpa fostering in me his love of nature, to now, being able to share the story of essential oils, I feel that Young Living has helped me fulfill a lifelong passion for better understanding the amazing and dynamic world of nature that God created.

Jason Smith

Royal Crown Diamond, Oklahoma

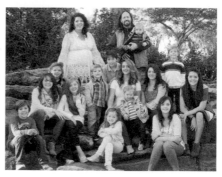

Young Living member since? 2009
Spouse: Christa Smith
Children: 15 (Ages 4 months to 20 years)
Hobbies: I play drums and bass guitar, and some guitar. And I enjoy researching economic and domestic and world events.

Favorite Young Living product? Akin to asking which of my children is my favorite, so my final answer is: whichever oil or supplement at that specific moment in time that I'm ingesting or smelling.

Favorite Young Living product gift? Anything that will promote a healthy immune system that will ultimately prolong or save their life!

Favorite Young Living farm or event? Convention, Europe convention and jousting at the farm in Mona. Oh and watching or helping distill any oil. Okay, that was 3 items really... basically about every farm and oil distillation and event. Oh, and of course the Diamond retreats and Leadership Cruise! Okay I'll stop now.

Describe your day using Young Living products:

Morning: A capful of orange oil, sometimes a cap of half Peppermint and half Ginger. Sometimes Ocotea, Cinnamon Bark and a cap of a few of my favorite oils for supporting the cardiovascular system. Usually AlkaLime, Super C, BLM and Sulfurzyme, one Nitro and NingXia Red packet, 1 or 2 swigs of MindWise, Thieves toothpaste, Young Living deodorant (the meadow one), Lavender shampoo, sometimes Essentialzyme, OmegaGize.

Afternoon: Before meals… Essentialzymes-4. And then whenever else... Essentialzyme: 2 to 4 caplets, ComforTone: 2 capsules. I will take ICP and sometimes another Nitro and a NingXia Red packet.

Evening: Stress Away, Peace & Calming, sometimes SleepEssence. Aroma Life, 2 Life 5 capsules, 1 or 2 swigs of MindWise, ComforTone: 2 caps, ICP, sometimes Detoxzyme, BLM and Sulfurzyme, Protec and Melaleuca Alternifolia (and I spelled that without looking it up but I'm pretty sure it's correct!)

What does Young Living mean to you? Freedom from the poison.

JD Hudgens

Diamond, Texas

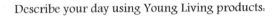

Young Living member since? June 2010
Spouse: Shannon Hudgens
Age: 39
Hobbies: CrossFit, computer programming
Favorite Young Living product?
NingXia Nitro

Favorite Young Living product to gift? It depends on the person and their needs.

Favorite Young Living farm or event? Yep, sure do love 'em all!

Describe your day using Young Living products:

Morning: NingXia Red and Nitro before shower. Peppermint during CrossFit workout. Thieves hand soap, Lavender shampoo, Meadow Mist deodorant, AromaBright toothpaste.

Afternoon: Thieves cleaner, Frankincense, Purification, Sulfurzyme, Longevity, Essentialzyme.

Evening: Lemon and Grapefruit in water. Joy and Valor over the heart. AromaSleep, Peace & Calming.

When traveling: Oh no! I forgot to put oils in my carry on! Grrr! Peppermint, Frankincense.

What does Young Living mean to you? Young Living is an entity that provides a path for people to find freedom in health, finances and time. For us, it transformed a fatherless home into a two parent household again and gave us an opportunity to share how we got here. God uses Young Living to bless people as we have seen first-hand.

What is your favorite clean eating meal? Glazed salmon, asparagus, sweet potatoes.

Jeanmarie Hepworth
Royal Crown Diamond, Colorado

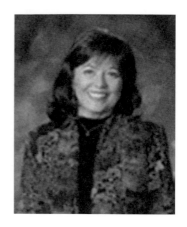

Young Living member since? 1992
Hobbies: Sewing, theater, reading, traveling
Favorite Young Living product?
Too many to list
Favorite Young Living product to gift? Many
Favorite Young Living farm or event?
Lavender Days and all the Young Living
Conventions

Describe your day using Young Living products:

Morning, Afternoon, & Evening: I have been using the Young Living product line for over 20 years and the products continue to provide me with a natural healthy lifestyle. I very seldom need to seek items outside of Young Living's product line as their personal care products, home products, animal care products, dietary products, and of course their essential oils have consistently proven to be superior. The familiar words often expressed among friends is "I have an Oil for that" and it is not a slight exaggeration in my world.

When Traveling: When preparing for a trip, my first thought turns to what essential oils and supplements I choose to have with me. It is as vitally important to me as the clothes I choose to pack.

What does Young Living mean to you? Young Living is my personal lifestyle, covering every aspect within my life, from physical, emotional, spiritual and financial well-being. Every day my life is richly filled in giving and sharing with others. It has brought me the gifts of friendship, community and extended family. Young Living has provided a way for me to share a gift that keeps on giving. I love witnessing the success these products have brought to thousands of other lives as well. I was blessed the day God changed my course of direction years ago and I have never looked back.

Jeffrey Lewis
Diamond, New York

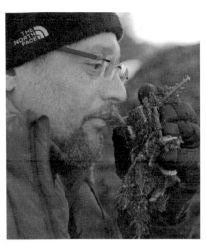

Young Living member since? 1997

Spouse: Gailann Greene

Age: 60

Hobbies: Travel, movies, basketball

Favorite Young Living product? NingXia Red, Lavender, DiGize & White Angelica

Favorite Young Living product to gift: NingXia Red

Favorite Young Living farm or event? Grand Convention and Diamond Trips

Describe your day using Young Living products:

Morning: Thieves AromaBright toothpaste and mouthwash. Put on: Valor, Harmony, Joy, White Angelica, Lavender, Shutran, Idaho Blue Spruce, Sacred Mountain followed by any oils that call to me for the day. Then I make a Power Meal smoothie with MindWise, Mineral Essence, JuvaPower, Sacred Frankincense, Ocotea, Copaiba and a ¼ bottle NingXia Red. Then take supplements: Super B & C, Prostate Health, Longevity, MultiGreens, OmegaGize and Essentialzyme. Diffuse oils at home and office.

Afternoon: Put on more oils like Frankincense, Harmony, Joy, White Angelica take Super B, Essentialzymes-4 & Essentialzyme, Ocotea, Sulfurzyme & BLM sometimes take Nitro. Use Thieves hand purifier a lot.

Evening: Life 5, ComforTone, Ocotea, Valor, Lavender, Geranium, Helichrysum, Prostate Health, Sulfurzyme, BLM, Genesis hand cream, Thieves hand purifier and spray. During the winter, I start taking Thieves lozenges throughout the day.

When Traveling: All oils mentioned above plus probably another 35 to 50 oils like all the Raindrop oils, Purification, DiGize, Thieves, Lemon, etc. Always bring enzymes and enough NingXia packets to take 3-4/day. Thieves spray & hand sanitizer, Allerzyme, Rehemogen, MindWise, all the supplements mentioned above.

What does Young Living mean to you? Young Living means healthy lifestyle, freedom, fun, great friendships and worldwide travel. It also means the ability to empower other's lives through sharing these products in a physical, spiritual & financial way.

What is your favorite clean eating meal? A field greens salad with grilled chicken.

Jennifer Breedlove

Gold, Missouri

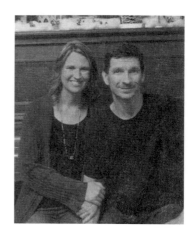

Young Living member since? August 2013
Spouse: Kevin Breedlove
Age: 38
Hobbies: Visiting National Parks across the USA, hiking with my family, reading a good book with a cup of hot tea
Favorite Young Living product? NingXia Red and Power Meal drink mix
Favorite Young Living product to gift? Lavender

Favorite Young Living farm or event? Silver Retreat

Describe your day using Young Living products:

Morning: Young Living Lavender shampoo, conditioner, and body wash in the shower. NingXia Red with breakfast. Power Meal shake for breakfast. Joy and Abundance on my heart.... Lemon in water before breakfast, Thieves toothpaste.
Afternoon: Citrus oils in my water all day, sometimes another Power Meal shake for lunch. Slique tea in the afternoon. Thieves hand soap. DIY deodorant with Young Living Purification oil. Young Living lip balm all day.
Evening: DIY foaming face wash with Frankincense and Orange. Thieves toothpaste, Thyromin, EndoGize, EndoFlex, True Source, Progessence Plus, Dragon Time, JuvaPower, Super B, AlkaLime, Super Cal, Sulfurzyme. Also Sandalwood face cream.

What does Young Living mean to you? Young Living's natural products enable me to take charge of my family's health. It gives me the tools to make wise choices that will equip us for our goals in all the areas of our life.

What is your favorite clean eating meal? Taco bowls... brown rice, seasoned chicken or beef, cheddar cheese, lettuce, tomato, salsa, black beans, avocado and sour cream.

Jennifer Jordan
Diamond, Kentucky

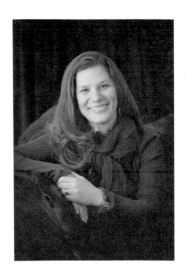

Young Living member since? 2009
Spouse: Adaryll Jordan
Age: 38
Hobbies: Reading, sewing, doing crazy things with my kids
Favorite Young Living product? NingXia Red, M-Grain and DiGize
Favorite Young Living farm or event? St. Maries Farm

Describe your day using Young Living products:

Morning: I use Lavender Mint shampoo and conditioner and shower gel with various oils. Then Satin Mint face scrub and the Orange Blossom face wash, Sandalwood moisturizer, Lavender lotion, Animal Scents ointment and Thieves oral care line. I use an Aria diffuser to diffuse Citrus Fresh. I use Awaken, EndoFlex, En-R-Gee, Lemon, Lavender, Peppermint, Copaiba, Grapefruit, Lemongrass, Marjoram, PanAway, Deep Relief, Believe, Motivation, and Oola infused oils. I also use NingXia Red, NingXia Nitro, Balance Complete, True Source, Sulfurzyme, CortiStop, MindWise, Super C, Essentialzyme, and MultiGreens.

Afternoon: M-Grain, Stress Away, Deep Relief, Valor, Thieves cleaner, Wolfberry bars!

Evening: NingXia Red, DiGize, Digest + Cleanse, Sulfurzyme, Essentialzyme, Multi-Greens, Cedarwood, Ortho Ease Massage Oil, bath salts made with Peace & Calming, Lavender or Stress Away.

When Traveling: I carry the everyday oils plus RC, DiGize, Copaiba, Breathe Again, Deep Relief, Oregano, Melrose, Helichrysum, Valor, Peace & Calming, and M-Grain everywhere I go. ImmuPower, Geranium, Mountain Savory, EndoFlex, En-R-Gee, Brain Power, Clarity, Raven, Palo Santo, Dorado Azul, Tea Tree, AromaEase, Dragon Time, Cedarwood and Citrus Fresh. I use a TheraPro diffuser when I travel.

What does Young Living mean to you? Freedom in my health. Freedom to educate myself and focus on wellness and what makes a body healthy. Freedom to empower others to experience the same. Financial freedom because of Young Living's generosity to pay me for sharing what I love with people I love. We now have the ability to give freely and provide our kids an opportunity to travel and see the world.

Jessica Gianelloni
Diamond, Louisiana

YL member since? 2013
Spouse: Rit Gianelloni
Age: 38
Hobbies: Orphans, Uganda, health, vaccine safety advocate
Favorite Young Living product?
Frankincense, Sheerlumé face cream, NingXia Red.

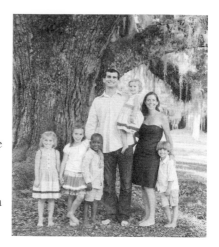

Favorite Young Living farm or event? The Sandalwood farm from the 2013 Drive to Win contest in Hawaii. I fell in love with the company on this trip!

Describe your day using Young Living products: What I love about Young Living is it has become a lifestyle for our entire family. With five small kids, I love that we all use Young Living products on a daily basis. My husband and kids each have their own routines. Here's mine:

Morning: Glass of NingXia Red with Frankincense, EndoFlex on my neck, Joy or a citrus oil in my diffuser, Peppermint in my coffee or tea (YUM), Life 5 probiotics and AlkaLime, Thieves laundry soap, Thieves dish soap, Hooray for the entire Thieves line!

Afternoon: Peppermint and Grapefruit or Lemon in my water, Frankincense inhaled and applied. NingXia Nitro for an afternoon boost. Something fabulous is always in the diffuser. One of my favorite combos is Frankincense, Lavender and Ylang Ylang.

Evening: I love the entire skin care line, specifically the Sheerlumé face cream, Boswellia Wrinkle Cream, and Wolfberry Eye Cream. Lavender or Release in the bath. Thieves toothpaste and mouthwash. Frankincense and Myrrh roll on across my face before bed. Tranquil on my feet. Nighty night!

When Traveling: Thieves internally, Oil on bottoms of feet. ImmuPower, Tranquil, Digest + Cleanse, and ParaFree (when traveling internationally).

What does Young Living mean to you? Wellness, Purpose and Abundance. This has been achieved in every aspect of our lives since joining Young Living: physically, spiritually, emotionally and financially. Young Living represents so much more than products. The Young Living Foundation is where my purpose and passion lives. Receiving the Spirit of the Foundation award is my greatest honor.

Jessica Laney Petty
Crown Diamond, California

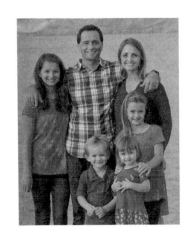

Young Living member since? 2013
Spouse: Nathan Petty
Age: 37
Hobbies: Helping at my kids' Waldorf school, traveling, reading
Favorite Young Living product? Thieves
Favorite Young Living farm or event?
Hawaiian Sandalwood Farm in Kona, Hawaii.

Describe your day using Young Living products:
Morning: Awaken, Envision, Joy, Live with Passion, Gratitude, Humility and many others. I brush my teeth with the AromaBright toothpaste. I take MultiGreens and Master Formula. I also often make a green smoothie with Balance Complete. *Afternoon:* There are oils all over my house including my kids' rooms, my office, the laundry room and my kitchen. I use them as needs arise. I also have other Young Liv- ing products throughout my house including diffusers and the Thieves Cleaner (in spray bottles) that I use in various rooms like my bathrooms and kitchen. I also carry oils, Young Living lip gloss and lip balm, Thieves Spray and Thieves Hand Sanitizer in my purse to use when I'm out.

Evening: In the evening I use Dream Catcher, Tranquil and Valor on my family to promote a restful night's sleep. I take Thyromin. I also use the ART skin care system at night and the Sandalwood Moisture Cream. I also brush my teeth with AromaBright, use the Thieves dental floss and mouthwash.

When Traveling: I use most of the same products in travel cases. I also am sure to bring lots of Thieves and ImmuPower to strengthen my family's immune systems. **What does Young Living mean to you?** In the last two years, Young Living has com- pletely changed my life. I think about our company about 90% of the time. I absolutely LOVE our products. I truly believe that a real passion for our products is the absolute KEY to success in this business. You have to love them so much that you would talk about them even if they weren't your business. You have to love sharing them with friends, family and new people you meet. That genuine passion has to shine through. It will draw people to you to learn more.

What is your favorite clean eating meal? I made a great salad last night with romaine lettuce, feta cheese, tomatoes, avocados, dressing and Taste of Italy essential oil.

Jihan Thomas
Diamond, New York

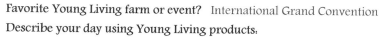

Young Living member since? 2004
Spouse: John Thomas
Age: 40
Hobbies: Oils!, walking, raw food, reading, leadership training, daydreaming.
Favorite Young Living product? Frankincense
Favorite Young Living product to gift? Abundance or NingXia

Favorite Young Living farm or event? International Grand Convention
Describe your day using Young Living products:
Morning: Thieves hand soap, toothpaste, Lavender shampoo, Lavender Mint conditioner, Mountain Mist deodorant, Valor, Abundance, Build Your Dream, NingXia Red, Mineral Essence, ART skin care system, ClaraDerm, Mint Satin Facial Scrub.... and so many more than I can think of!!
Afternoon: NingXia Red, several oils including Frankincense, Inspiration, Stress Away, Lavender, Abundance, Peppermint, or whatever else I'm drawn to.
Evening: I will take NingXia Nitro if I am going to be out (I usually go to bed early), Roman Chamomile, Super C, Thyromin, Allerzyme and Super Cal.

What does Young Living mean to you? I always say that Young Living does not define me, and it doesn't, but I am fully engrossed in the Young Living lifestyle. It has helped my family and I maintain awesome health and has given us the financial freedom and peace of mind to focus on what is important to us. We get to spend a lot of family time together, are gradually paying off all of our debts (including our student loans and mortgage), are traveling more, etc. With Young Living, we get to experience life in a whole different way than the average person stuck in the daily grind and for that we are forever grateful. Being in a business model where we can share this full lifestyle with others is what brings a whole new level of purpose to our lives and keeps us going. "Blessing" is an understatement!

What is your favorite clean eating meal? I love food, especially raw food and shakes. Anything with avocado and anything I can put in the blender makes me happy. Oh and pizza... and chocolate... but they're not clean. Ha!

Jilene Hay
Diamond, Canada

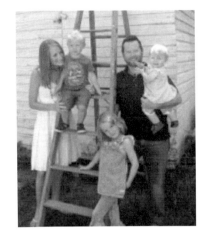

Young Living member since? January 2012
Spouse: Duane Hay
Age: Early 30's
Hobbies: Traveling, biking, exploring, enjoying good food
Favorite Young Living product? ART line
Favorite Young Living farm or event?
Winter Harvest at the Highland Flats Farm

Describe your day using Young Living products:

Morning: Shot of NingXia Red, MultiGreens and OmegaGize. We'll also make a smoothie with Balance Complete or Pure Protein Complete. We often make the Einkorn pancakes, as they kids LOVE them! ART Foaming Cleanser or Orange Blossom facial wash (I filled up an empty ART Cleanser bottle with ½ facial wash and ½ water and it works perfect!). We buy the Young Living bath and shower gel base and add in our own oils to it. I only wash my hair about 2 times a week but I love the Lavender Mint shampoo and conditioner. I use DIY deodorant and add Ylang Ylang and other oils. We all use AromaBright toothpaste. I use the ART toner and Sheerlumé. We also have Thieves hand soap.

Afternoon: Another shot of NingXia Red and MultiGreens. I will usually throw in a couple packages of NingXia for the kids wherever we go. We run the diffuser, we clean up using Thieves cleaner pretty much everywhere: floors, counters, laundry, etc. We LOVE the hand soap to help tackle any stains on the kids' clothes!

Evening: Fill kid's diffusers. In our bedroom, I love diffusing Idaho Balsam Fir. At night, everyone gets a Life 5 and oily feet. My personal favorite is RutaVaLa. I will often have a bath with some Epsom salts mixed with Lavender and Valor. My bedtime facial routine includes the ART foaming cleanser, toner and moisturizer.

What does Young Living mean to you? Young Living has been such a blessing in our lives! It has given me purpose and ignited the passion within me. I LOVE being able to share such amazing products coupled with a powerful opportunity to really impact and change people's lives. Young Living has given us an opportunity to speak life into people around us and empower others to see their full potential on every level – physically, emotionally and spiritually. We love seeing families come together and believe that Young Living is a gift to help families really thrive in all aspects of life.

Jill Young
Crown Diamond, New York

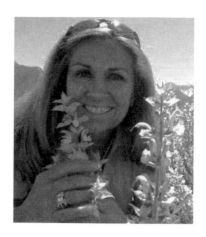

Young Living member since? 1996
Spouse: James Young
Age: 56
Hobbies: Traveling, gardening
Favorite Young Living product? MultiGreens
Favorite Young Living product to gift?
Abundance oil
Favorite Young Living farm or event?
St. Maries Farm in Idaho

Describe your day using Young Living products:

Morning: I start my day with Valor, Harmony and Abundance oil. Supplements include Essentialzyme, MultiGreens, Nitro & NingXia Red. Often I will switch up with Super Cal, Comfortone and ICP.

Afternoon: OmegaGize, Essentialzyme and MindWise. I also use Lime, Grapefruit and Lemon in water throughout the day.

Evening: In the evenings, I will use White Angelica oil, Geranium, Magnify Your Purpose, Peace & Calming as well as AlkaLime, Life 5 and Detoxzyme and Longevity capsules. Then I'll apply Lavender lotion, Orange Blossom facial wash and Sheerlumé.

When Traveling: Thieves oil, hand sanitizer, Essentialzyme, MultiGreens, Detoxzyme and Inner Defense

What does Young Living mean to you? How can you put into words the gratitude you feel when you have found your life's purpose and passion in a company that not only gives you better health, but a family of friends from around the world? There is no greater opportunity to help someone better his or her life and Young Living provides that for everybody who gives it a chance. Young Living is my lifestyle of choice! This company has made me the person I am today. Not better than anyone else, just better than I used to be in every way! I truly cannot imagine my life without these precious little drops of God in every bottle. Thank you Gary and Mary Young for the wellness, purpose and abundance you share with the world!

What is your favorite clean eating meal? Salad with fresh mixed greens, seeds and nuts!

Joanne Kan
Royal Crown Diamond, Hong Kong

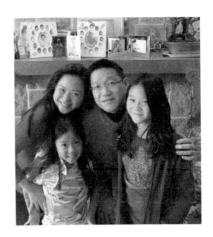

Young Living member since? 2011
Spouse: Eric Yang
Age: 44
Hobbies: Read, play with my oils, Ted Talks
Favorite Young Living product? Awaken oil
Favorite Young Living farm or event?
The winter harvest!

Describe your day using Young Living products:

Morning: In the mornings I will use the ART face wash (or Orange Blossom), toner and serum with Sandalwood oil (or Sheerlumé), AromaBright Toothpaste, NingXia Red and Mineral Essence. I also take MegaCal, Sulfurzyme, Super B, MultiGreens, OmegaGize, CortiStop/Thyromin, Essentialzyme, Balance Complete, ICP, JuvaPower, and AlkaLime. Now I'm doing Highest Potential, Motivation and Sacred Mountain. If I go out, I use Neroli + Rose as perfume. I love White Angelica, Harmony, Joy and Valor or Valor II. This really helps me stay positive. I will use Magnify Your Purpose, Transformation and Believe sometimes. If I need them, I use Acceptance or Surrender.

Afternoon: NingXia Red. To overcome obstacles: Feelings Kit. L' Brianté lip gloss. If I am teaching, I always put on Common Sense, Clarity and Magnify Your Purpose, drink a Nitro and NingXia. If I'm tired: Brain Power. I also spray the room with Common Sense, Acceptance and Believe. I shower using Young Living's shower gel, shampoo and conditioner. I also use a homemade sugar scrub. I use Thieves cleaner often.

Evening: I will take AlkaLime, Ocotea, Sulfurzyme, Detoxzyme, Essentialzymes-4 and Grapefruit oil in capsules. Cel-Lite Massage oil, JuvaCleanse & Citrus Fresh as body oil, OrthoEase on shoulders, lower back & lower legs. I take Inner Defense often after work. I drop Raindrop oils on my feet after I get in bed.

What does Young Living mean to you? It's not about just rubbing on a few oils. It's about understanding what is good for us—diet, lifestyle and making the right choices. It's about inspiring people around us to do the same. It's about being the best we can; self-development, character building. And we have the best tool to do that because the oils work! Through all of this, we achieve purpose and abundance not only for ourselves but for those who are inspired to get on board with us to walk this amazing journey together. It is PRICELESS to see those people transform.

Jodi McKenna

Diamond, Indiana

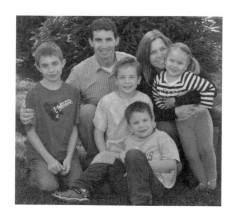

Young Living member since? 2007
Spouse: Brian McKenna
Age: 39
Hobbies: I love to date my husband, make homemade almond milk, curl up with a good book, backpack into the mountains, watch movies and spend time with my kids, and do Pilates reformer.

Favorite Young Living product? Frankincense and Black Spruce
Favorite Young Living product to gift? Cool Azul
Favorite Young Living farm or event? Spring planting at Highland Flats

Describe your day using Young Living products:

Morning: My day typically begins with Valor, Joy, Harmony and White Angelica. Depending on how I am feeling, I might add Frankincense or Patchouli to my neck. I drink NingXia Red with Lemon and Orange essential oil. I take Super C chewable tablet as my morning candy. The diffuser is loaded with an oil specific to our day.

Afternoon: You will often find me loading the kitchen diffuser with Believe or Clarity and drinking a NingXia Red shot with Nitro. I often take Longevity and my Multi-Greens for sustained energy.

Evening: To support that lovely thing called sleep, I take OmegaGize before bedtime along with Life 5. Oh, and I love me some Clary Sage and Progessence Plus before the lights go out! Who knows, the Ylang Ylang sometimes makes and appearance too.

What does Young Living mean to you? I love that Young Living stands for Wellness, Purpose and Abundance. Young Living is my calling. I know that I that the Lord called me to work within Young Living to share about the tools and resources that God left for us on earth—plants that have been here since He made them. I love teaching people about essential oils through scripture and then equipping people to use oil infused products confidently within their homes and at their friend's homes.

Jodie Vickers
Gold, Missouri

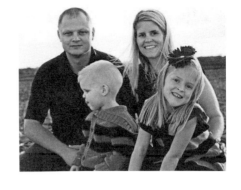

Young Living member since? June 2013
Spouse: Ryan Vickers
Age: 35
Hobbies: Reading, camping, teaching and serving others
Favorite Young Living product? Thieves
Favorite Young Living product to gift?
I have gifted many oils depending on the need

Describe your day using Young Living products:

Morning: Lavender shampoo and conditioner, Thieves AromaBright toothpaste, Frankincense and coconut oil for face moisturizer, Master Formula supplement, True Source vitamins, shot of NingXia, Joy over my heart, Progessence Plus on my wrists, and Believe behind my ears.
Afternoon: NingXia Nitro, Stress Away, Thieves cleaner
Evening: Cedarwood for encouraging a restful night's sleep, we diffuse Sleepyize for the kids, oils on feet for everyone!

What does Young Living mean to you? Since becoming a member of Young Living in 2013, I can honestly say this company has forever changed the way I look at health and wellness! Young Living and their products have empowered me as a mother, wife and teacher! Every time I use my oils or natural products to help my friends and family have a more chemical free home, I can't help but be amazed and thankful at God's design in nature.

What is your favorite clean eating meal? Chicken salad is my favorite "clean" meal, but honestly this is one area my family is working on! We are a work in progress! We are definitely moving in the right direction though!

Jordan Schrandt

Crown Diamond, Missouri

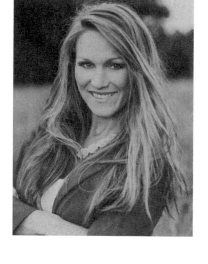

Young Living member since? 2012
Spouse: Doug Schrandt
Age: 28
Hobbies: Running, working out, writing, event planning, speaking, traveling, gardening, family activities, homesteading, cooking, being involved with church and playing the piano
Favorite Young Living product? Nitro
Favorite Young Living product to gift?
Thieves home products
Favorite Young Living farm or event?
Drive to Win 2014 in Hawaii
Describe your day using Young Living products:

Morning: ART skin care line, SheerLume, and sometimes the ART masque on my face. I alternate between all the shampoos and conditioners. I always take OmegaGize, Multigreens, Longevity, Super C, and Master Formula every day. I diffuse various oils but I really love Clarity and Believe. We use all the Thieves products and I love diffusing oils during our homeschool time. Usually I take a capsule of a citrus oil, Myrrh and Lemongrass. I drink Protein Complete as part of my breakfast.

Afternoon: Throughout the day I am constantly rubbing on different oils. I will grab various oils from my oil bag and use them before and after most activities. I really love drinking Nitro all through the day, too.

Evening: I take the same supplements in the evening. I love putting Animal Scents ointment on my feet before bed. I often use Ylang Ylang, Geranium and Rose before bed. I also love Lavender lotion, a DIY deodorant spray and the Thieves toothpaste.

What does Young Living mean to you? The Young Living lifestyle has changed my life in almost every way possible. I love eating clean and having a chemical free home. I love protecting my family from toxic junk... it is incredibly empowering! I love Young Living and the products they provide... and I love the opportunity to share that lifestyle with people around the world!

Julie Hosman

Silver, Missouri

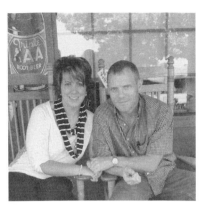

Young Living member since? 2013

Spouse: Jason Hosman

Hobbies: Kids: dance, piano and football… just going to all their stuff. I research oils and products and emotional health all the time

Favorite Young Living product? NingXia Red

Favorite Young Living product to gift? Cinnamint Lip Balm

Favorite Young Living farm or event? Silver Retreat

Describe your day using Young Living products:

Morning: Thieves tooth paste and mouthwash, MultiGreens, lots of NingXia Red, MindWise, NingXia Nitro, Master Formula, and a drop of Joy over my heart. I also wear Abundance as a perfume.

Afternoon: We diffuse En-R-Gee, Lime or Abundance. I love using Orange oil. Also I'm in love with Thieves cleaner in every room of the house and the whole Thieves line for home care and on-the-go, too! I love diffusing fall scents during fall months, Christmas scents around the holidays, light clean scents in the spring, and fun outdoorsy scents in summer!

Evening: I take MultiGreens and Master Formula again. I love to use Tranquil in the evenings and diffuse Peace & Calming (1 or 2). Also Orange or Lavender are favorites before bed. I always use the Young Living ART line for my face, Lavender lotion, and my favorite shampoo and conditioner is Lavender Mint.

What does Young Living mean to you? Young Living has absolutely changed my life. It's made me aware of all the toxins I had in my home. It's one of the main reasons I've learned about the emotional side of using oils, which sets captives free! My family is happier and healthier now more than ever.

What is your favorite clean eating meal? Grilled chicken with Lemon oil, broccoli and a sweet potato.

Karen Douglas
Diamond, Texas

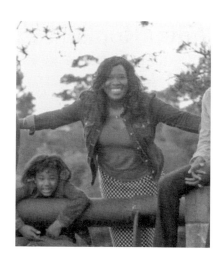

YL member since? 2002

Age: 49

Hobbies: Hangout with my children (I think they are so cool), shopping, walking, camping, sports, entrepreneurship, homeschooling my children.

Favorite Young Living product?
Boswellia Wrinkle Cream

Favorite Product to Gift? Peppermint oil

Favorite Young Living farm or event? International Grand Convention

Describe your day using Young Living products:

Morning: I start my day by using ART Skin Care System along with the ART Serum for a clean, fresh, moisturized feeling. I then add a few drops of Lemon to my water to quench my thirst. Supplements: JuvaTone, Master Formula, Sulfurzyme, BLM, Longevity, Super C, Super B, MultiGreens, Allerzyme, Essentialzyme, 3 ounces of NingXia Red with two drops of Peppermint, Thieves, Oregano and a Nitro combined. Dental Care: Thieves AromaBright toothpaste, mouthwash and floss. Deodorant: Thieves Dentarome Toothpaste (YES, toothpaste for deodorant) Oils: Valor on my spine, Joy over my heart, Abundance on my forearms, Common Sense, Brain Power, RC, Copaiba, Magnify Your Purpose, Oola Balance with one of the Oola "F" oils, White Angelica, Progessence Plus. I use Lavender lotion all day.

Afternoon: Supplements: Allerzyme, Essentialzyme, Sulfurzyme, BLM, Super C, Multi-Greens, NingXia Red, Nitro (sometimes). Oils: Thieves, Stress Away, Ocotea, Peppermint, Breathe Again, Progessence Plus.

Evening: Supplements: Same as morning but add Life 5. Oils: Longevity oil, Frankincense, Myrrh, Tea Tree, Cedarwood, EndoFlex, ImmuPower, DiGize, Progessence Plus. ART Skin Care System, ART serum, Boswellia Wrinkle Cream, Wolfberry Eye Cream, Evening Shower Gel. AromaBright toothpaste, Thieves mouthwash and floss. Thieves Household Cleaner all over and in wiper fluid in cars.

What does Young Living mean to you? The Lord placed Young Living in our lives when we needed it the most! Whether it was to enhance our immune system or support our family financially, these stellar oils have given us a new lease on life!

Karen Hopkins

Royal Crown Diamond, Oklahoma

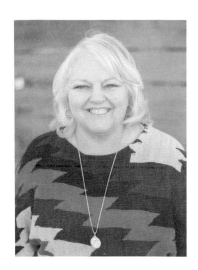

Young Living member since? July 2006

Spouse: Max Hopkins

Age: 62

Hobbies: Coin collecting

Favorite Young Living product?

NingXia Red and Nitro

Favorite Young Living farm or event?

Grand Convention

Describe your day using Young Living products:

Morning: 2 Nitro, 4-6 ounces NingXia Red in filtered water. 6 full dropper squirts of Mineral Essence in water bottle with 10 drops each of Slique Essence and Grapefruit. Mixture or full capsules of Copaiba, Juva Cleanse and DiGize. Inner Defense; several enzymes; Essentialzyme, Sulfurzyme, and MightyZyme (I love to chew something after so many capsules). Throughout the day I take Thyromin and BLM. I take AlkaLime after walking. Then ART skin line, Wolfberry Eye Cream, Thieves AromaBright tooth-paste, Lavender shampoo and conditioner.

Afternoon: I use Thieves and Exodus II throughout the day on my gums, but especially after eating to keep my teeth looking white and cleaner. 30 minutes after eating, I take full capsules of Ocotea, Coriander, Fennel, Dill, Cinnamon and Thieves.

Evening: I take MultiGreens and Life 5 at night. I usually take my morning oils again before my head hits the pillow if it is before 11:00 p.m. If later than that, I rub Myrrh and Myrtle over my thyroid. I take 10 Detoxzyme late at night.

What does Young Living mean to you? My daughter, Sera Johnson, introduced me to Debra Raybern who helped me understand how essential oils worked with my body systems. I've only used Young Living Essential Oils since they are a pure therapeutic grade. I was a former Home Economics teacher that was morbidly obese. I felt that the Lord Jesus was asking me to start a Daniel fast (mostly vegetables), which seemed im-possible since I was addicted to sugar. I tried many different dieting programs in the past, but nothing worked on a long time basis. I started ingesting several oils that help support the blood system. It was amazing! I also noticed that the more YLEOs that I ingested, the more my appetite was under control.

Karen Vavrick
Diamond, Michigan

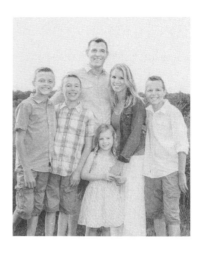

Young Living member since? August 2013
Spouse: Paul Vavrick
Age: 35
Hobbies: Yoga, exercising, Bible studying, helping out in my daughter's classroom, watching my boys play sports, traveling
Favorite Young Living product? NingXia Red
Favorite Young Living product to gift? Thieves Cleaner

Describe your day using Young Living products:

Morning: I always start my morning diffusing—usually Citrus Fresh with a few others. Peppermint helps me wake up and get moving, and the citrus oils boost our mood. We call them our "happy" oils. We all take a shot glass of NingXia Red after breakfast as well. My husband and I take Longevity after breakfast as well. I take BLM as I've had a lifetime of knee issues and surgeries for joint health. My husband and I also take Master Formula multi-vitamins.

Afternoon: In the afternoon I'm usually diffusing something uplifting or cleansing like Thieves, Purification, Motivation, Lime, Joy, etc. It really depends on the day and what I'm doing and trying to accomplish. I apply oils topically as needed. When my kids arrive home from school I always diffuse Thieves to clean the air and any hitchhikers they may have brought with them, and Valor is really helpful to diffuse during homework time. We also take Life 5 probiotic at some point in the afternoon.

Evening: I take MultiGreens, Super C, as well as Inner Defense (taken as needed, not regularly). We have diffusers going in each bedroom. Everyone has their favorites to diffuse at night - some being Dream Catcher, Valor, Lavender, Peace & Calming. Before I go to bed, I use the ART skincare system and add a drop of Frankincense in the face cream, as well as the Wolfberry eye cream. We use Thieves toothpastes, mouthwash, and floss. We also love all of Young Living's shampoos and conditioners. Tranquil and RutaVaLa roll ons are always on our nightstand bedside as well.

What does Young Living mean to you? Young Living means a life of health and wellness for my family, and freedom to work the hours we want, travel the world, and help people pursue their dreams of the same.

Karla Berger
Diamond, Minnesota

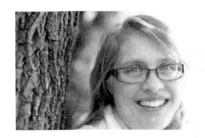

Young Living member since? 2001

Spouse: David Berger

Age: 54

Hobbies: Travel (especially overseas) and spending time with my family

Favorite Young Living product? NingXia Red

Favorite Young Living product to gift? Peppermint Oil or NingXia Red

Favorite Young Living farm or event? The Ecuador Farm

Describe your day using Young Living products:

Morning: NingXia Red, Mineral Essence, Thyromin, OmegaGize, Nitro, Balance Complete, or Pure Protein, MultiGreens, Motivation or Believe oil, (or Envision for business support) and Aroma Life.

Afternoon: Slique Tea, Nitro

Evening: NingXia Red, Thyromin, OmegaGize, MultiGreens, MegaCal, Cedarwood, ComforTone, Sulfurzyme, Aroma Life.

When Traveling: OmegaGize, Thyromin, NingXia Red, Nitro, all the oils from the Everyday oils kit.

What does Young Living mean to you? In one word, Young Living to us means FREEDOM! Within a week of using the Young Living oils, we knew it was a "fit"! What we didn't know is how we would be able to pay for our new love. We had just had our eighth baby and we were going further into debt every month as we were striving to live on one meager income. Thankfully, Young Living provided a way for us to not only purchase the products we loved, but to impact others' lives and experience financial abundance and freedom beyond our expectations.

What is your favorite clean eating meal? I love variety so making fruit and veggie smoothies is my ideal clean eating. I love to throw in greens, fruit, some Balance Complete or Pure Protein and an essential oil or two to change up the flavor!

Kate Haymes

Silver, Missouri

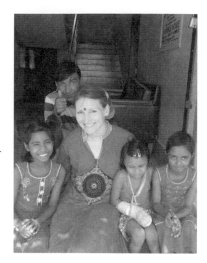

Young Living member since? 2013

Spouse: Not yet!

Age: 27

Hobbies: Flying airplanes, Bible studying, learning, exercising, traveling, serving, being with lively people!

Favorite Young Living product? Tie between NingXia Red and Wolfberry Crisp bars!

Favorite Young Living product to gift? Whatever I think they would most benefit

Describe your day using Young Living products:

Morning: I start my morning brushing with AromaBright toothpaste then I use the ART line (which I really like!). The Lavender shampoo and conditioner are shower essentials. I take a little more than one ounce of NingXia Red as communion juice most mornings, Master Formula and depending on the day and the need, I take a capsule full of varying oils, with citrus oils almost always being part of that blend.

Afternoon: For my typical day, items in the Thieves line get good use around the home and on the go. I have several oils in a spray bottles mixed with filtered water in my purse and around the house. I also apply several oils topically throughout the day with some favorites being Harmony, Peppermint, and any of the citrus oils. Nitro often.

Evening: In the evening I use my diffuser, often with Lavender, but that varies. I love applying oils neat to my feet at night. Typically Thieves is one of the oils I apply. Before I go to bed, I use the same morning facial regimen, except I also like to put oils on my face before moisturizing. I like Frankincense, Lavender, Melrose and Tea Tree, varying what I use each time. I use Thieves AromaBright toothpaste at night as well.

When Traveling: My travel bag of oils and supplements has been helpful on mission trips for myself and others and includes: Frankincense, Melrose, Lemon, Harmony, Purification, Thieves, Clove, RC, Lavender, Peppermint, DiGize and Stress Away.

What does Young Living mean to you? I believe in working hard for a purpose you are passionate about. Young Living's mission to steward creation, create a community where healing and learning collide, and inspire people to wellness, purpose and abundance in every area goes hand in hand with God's intention for His beloved creation!

Kathy Farmer

Royal Crown Diamond, Colorado

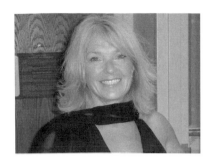

Young Living member since? October 1993

Spouse: Mark McCaskill

Age: ...we are Young Living after all!

Hobbies: Reading, connecting with friends, traveling.

Favorite Young Living product? Sacred Frankincense, NingXia Red and Nitro.

Favorite Young Living farm or event? Diamond trips in Thailand and Oman.

Describe your day using Young Living products:

Morning: We start the day with AlkaLime. Sometimes with our schedule we eat too late to take it at night, so we always take it in the morning. Then Mark and I put oils on each other...on the back, along the spine especially. It varies, but we always use things like Frankincense and Idaho Balsam Fir. Usually by the time we are done we have used about 15 oils or so. Then we will take NingXia Red. I am a master herbalist, so we most often mix some liquid herbs into our NingXia. We also use Thieves toothpaste and mouthwash. Before I put on my make up, I use my Progessence Plus and ART. I do PD 80/20, Cortistop and EndoGize and I personally like to take them in the morning when I take Essentialzymes-4: before breakfast.

Afternoon: Nitro is used throughout the day. I take Inner Defense or Longevity as I think of it. Between meals I like to take Detoxzyme. Most days we use a lot of Copaiba, Helichrysum and Sacred Frankincense.

Evening: At the end of the day we LOVE Epsom salt baths with Evening Peace or Sensation Bath & Shower Gel.

What does Young Living mean to you? We live a Young Living lifestyle. It is who I am. I love how people always say how great I smell (just happened 2 nights ago at a restaurant and I hadn't put on oils for hours!) Our energy levels are through the roof...and if I feel it dragging a bit, a Nitro gets me back on track! I love that we can entertain house guests from around the world! We are all part of a global Young Living family...nothing could be more awesome! We love being able to share that ability!

Kathy Kouwe

Crown Diamond, New York

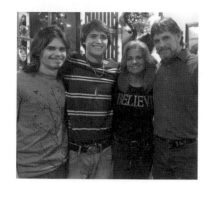

Young Living member since? 1996
Spouse: Chip Kouwe
Age: 52
Hobbies: Riding my motorcycle
Favorite Young Living product?
It depends on the day
Favorite Young Living product to gift? Joy
Favorite Young Living farm or event? Working at the St. Maries Lavender Harvest many years ago

Describe your day using Young Living products:

Morning: I put Peppermint on my head and inhale. Brush with AromaBright. I use Thyromin, CortiStop, and take NingXia Red, a tablespoon of MindWise, a Nitro, Mineral Essence, Essentialzyme, OmegaGize, Sulfurzyme, BLM, MultiGreens, Longevity, JuvaTone, wash face with ART facial cleanser, Sheerlumé or Sandalwood.

Afternoon: Essentialzymes-4, Detoxzyme, sometimes ComforTone, many oils… whatever I am sharing or in the mood for. We are always diffusing many oils.

Evening: I like all the bath gels and soaps so I alternate them all. Copaiba shampoo and conditioner is my favorite. After my bath (that has oils in it), Valor on the feet & shoulders, Harmony on the chakras, Joy over my heart and ears, Release over the liver, Frankincense and Lavender over the chest and abdomen, White Angelica on the shoulders, EndoFlex on thyroid & lower back then Lavender, Genesis or Sensation lotion. I enjoy using all the facial products. I alternate Life 5, SleepEssence and if I'm feeling I need more: BLM and Sulfurzyme.

What does Young Living mean to you? Young Living is my life. It's not what I do; it's who I am. Young Living has given me a passion with a purpose that I never dreamed I would have. Young Living has given me a new family and so many friendships worldwide as well as my health, a healthy family and so much freedom. I truly believe Young Living has helped me achieve the best health and wellness I've ever had!

Kelli Wright
Crown Diamond, Alabama

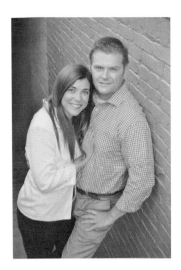

Young Living member since? 2012

Spouse: Les Wright

Age: 38

Hobbies: Antiques, estate sales, yard sales, decorating, being crafty, photography and hanging out with my family!

Favorite Young Living product? How in the world do you pick just one? I guess if I have to: NingXia!

Favorite Young Living farm or event?
Oh my goodness, they have all been so wonderful. I think the most memorable trip was Silver Retreat in Spokane and Saint Maries.

Describe your day using Young Living products:

Morning: I wake up and drink NingXia Red right away. Then for breakfast I use the Balance Complete to make a smoothie full of fruit and green goodness! I wash my face with ART cleanser and moisturize with argan oil and whatever oil I am in the mood for that day! It could be Myrrh, Geranium, Frankincense or Ylang Ylang.

Afternoon: Sometimes if I am super slammed, I down another Balance Complete shake. I take Nitro for an added pick-me-up. Most days you will find me inhaling some Stress Away or bathing in the Stress Away roll on. I also use Esssetialzymes-4 after meals.

Evening: I take BLM for my muscles, OmegaGize, Sulfurzyme, Master Formula, Thyromin and then Life 5 and I am off to bed!

What does Young Living mean to you? Young Living has changed our lives for the better in so many ways. I always tell people all the time, and I am serious... even if I didn't make a dime off of these products I would still use them and shout them from the rooftops: they are that awesome! We have been using Young Living products for three years and our health has never been better. The Young Living lifestyle is really a way of life for us. We are so much more mindful of what we are putting in and on our bodies, making sure that we live as chemical free as possible. Not only is our health better than ever for it, but we have also been able to share our lifestyle with others who have seen the same incredible results. We have been able to create a full-time income doing something that we are passionate about and we are so grateful!

Kelly Rigterink
Silver, Michigan

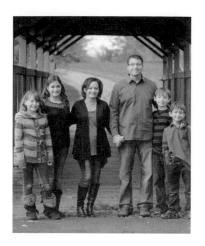

Young Living member since? September 2013
Spouse: Ryan Rigterink
Hobbies: Traveling, game nights with family and friends
Favorite Young Living product? NingXia Red
Favorite Young Living product to gift? I love to give Lavender or Thieves
Favorite Young Living farm or event? Mona, Utah. It was incredible to be a part of the Seed to Seal process!

Describe your day using Young Living products:

Morning: When I get up I drink a few ounces of water with 3-4 drops of Lemon and 1-2 ounces of NingXia Red. I use Lavender Mint shampoo and conditioner, DIY body wash with essential oils (currently Joy) and Citrus Fresh Sugar Scrub. I will also use Meadow Mist Deodorant, Thieves toothpaste (my mouth has never been happier), ART moisturizer, EndoFlex, a drop of Joy on my heart, Thieves, and a capsule of whatever oils I feel would be of benefit. I take AlkaLime most days. Sulfurzyme is a must, Super C, Master Formula, MultiGreens.

Afternoon: I will take Nitro in the afternoon if I am in a slump. Thieves hand soap is by every sink. I also use Thieves cleaner in the kitchen and bathrooms.

Evening: I use Progessence Plus, Tranquil and Thyromin at night.

When Traveling: Thieves spray, diffuser with Thieves or Purification, Thieves hand purifier, NingXia Red, most of my oils go with me.

What does Young Living mean to you? Young Living has been such an unexpected blessing! Over the past 10-15 years it has been a growing passion of mine to support my family's wellness as naturally as possible. Young Living came into the picture two years ago and it has helped us to take a giant leap forward purging toxins out of our home and learning what things to use to support our bodies best. Not only that, but I have been blessed with incredible friendships and comradery. I never intended to do the business side, but it happened naturally as people saw the benefits we experienced.

What is your favorite clean eating meal? Taco Salad made with organic greens, tomatoes, beans, grass fed beef seasoned with homemade seasoning and garden salsa. Yum!

Kendra Pope

Executive, Pennsylvania

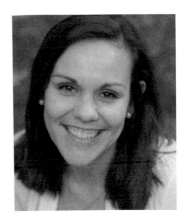

Young Living member since? September 2014

Spouse: Timotheus Pope

Age: 32

Hobbies: Spending time with my husband and kids, working out, reading, blogging.

Favorite Young Living product? NingXia Nitro

Favorite Young Living product to gift? NingXia Nitro

Describe your day using Young Living products:

Morning: Thieves toothpaste to brush, Nitro pre-workout, NingXia Red post-workout. Lavender Mint shampoo and conditioner on my hair and Joy on my wrists and on my diffuser necklace!

Afternoon: Diffusing whatever oils I'm in the mood for that day, usually something uplifting and energizing like a citrus and mint or En-R-Gee. We wash our hands all day long with DIY Thieves hand soap. I mop and clean surfaces with Thieves cleaner.

Evening: Diffuse something relaxing and rub RutaVaLa roll on for my temples and on most nights get a shoulder rub with Relaxation massage oil.

When Traveling: I take my most used oils with me in a case everywhere I go! Thieves, Lavender, Peppermint, Joy, Lemon, RC and DiGize to be specific. Also my Thieves toothpaste and Lavender Mint shampoo and conditioner.

What does Young Living mean to you? Young Living means a better quality of life and health to me. I don't have to worry about the everyday products I'm using hurting me or my family's bodies and that is SUCH a relief. It means natural products that I can trust and a safer home for my family.

What is your favorite clean eating meal? We love a HUGE salad of different greens with chicken, fruit, nuts and olive oil and vinegar to top it!

Krista Haymes

Platinum, Missouri

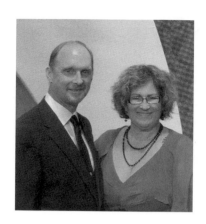

Young Living member since? 2013

Spouse: Jason Haymes

Age: 53

Children: Lindsay Haymes, Jordan Schrandt, Kate Haymes and Seth Haymes.

Hobbies: Traveling, being with family, learning

Favorite Young Living product? Valor

Favorite Young Living farm or event? Salt Lake City Convention

Describe your day using Young Living products:

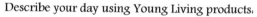

Morning: I take NingXia Red, Super C chewable, Longevity and a variety of oils in a capsule or two with water. Sometimes I have warm water with a few drops of Lemon oil. I use Orange Blossom Facial Wash and Sandalwood Cream.

Afternoon: I apply or take various oils throughout the day. I LOVE Rose Ointment! I take several Sulfurzyme capsules throughout the day and after meals. Occasionally, I drink Slique tea or a NingXia Nitro for a pick me up! I use Thieves cleaner throughout day as needed. In the laundry room, I have a wool dryer ball and drop a few drops of Purification, which I use to replace dryer sheets! These products are totally integrated into our world!

Evening: I take Life 5 with water and diffuse oils at night. Putting oils on my pillow is key to a good, restful night's sleep and will also support my body systems and creativity. Some that are especially helpful are Dream Catcher and Highest Potential. If my immune system needs support I will put oils on the bottoms of my feet.

What does Young Living mean to you? Discovering Young Living has opened my eyes to a whole new paradigm of health and wellness! I love Gary Young for his sincere, down to earth, spiritual approach to creating these amazing products for us! I love Young Living and want to share the message of the Seed to Seal calling with everyone! It's liberating to totally trust products that not only "detox" but also "don't tox" to begin with! Bringing Young Living into every home in the world is an honorable effort and I'm so excited to be a part!

What is your favorite clean eating meal? Grass fed, clean beef from our family farm, homegrown vegetables and farm fresh milk from our neighbors' dairy!

Ladonna Beals
Diamond, Oklahoma

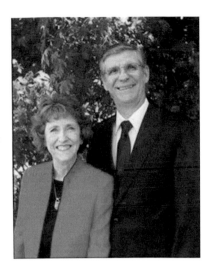

Young Living member since? November 2009
Spouse: Terry Beals
Age: 61
Hobbies: Reading, sugar free and wheat free cooking
Favorite Young Living product? NingXia Red
Favorite Young Living product to gift?
Lavender lotion
Favorite Young Living farm or event?
Love all the farms; the retreats are priceless!

Describe your day using Young Living products:

Morning: I drink NingXia Red and a Nitro mixed with 6 ounces or more water and some Orange oil. I take Thyromin, EndoGize, OmegaGize, Sulfurzyme, Longevity, BLM and Essentialzymes-4. I take a few capsules of oils and that varies with the season. In the spring, I was taking Lemon and DiGize and now I am taking GLF. I use Lavender bath gel and either Lavender or Copaiba Vanilla shampoo and conditioner. I use ART skin care on my face and Boswellia Wrinkle cream or Sheerlumé. Most used oils: Aroma Life, Copaiba, Frankincense, Joy and Progessence Plus. DiGize after eating.

Afternoon: More Essentialzyme or Essentialzymes-4 and DiGize after lunch. Usually have a glass of AlkaLime sometime in the middle of the afternoon. Around 3, I repeat my NingXia and Nitro blend that I did in the morning. After every meal or snack, I wipe my sinks and counters down with Thieves Household Cleaner. Every time we change our sheets, I spray the mattress and pillows with Thieves. I also add Thieves to laundry that needs a boost and I use wool dryer balls sprayed with Thieves.

Evening: More Essentialzymes-4, Detoxzyme, ComforTone, ART skin care. After showering, I use Genesis lotion and more Boswellia Wrinkle cream and Sheerlumé.

What does Young Living mean to you? I truly believe that Young Living is a gift from God to me. First, the products elevated me to a new level of wellness and second they have allowed us financial freedom better than we ever hoped or imagined possible. By the time we were Gold, our Young Living income surpassed my husband's pastor salary significantly. We especially enjoy the freedom to give to others from the abundance the LORD has given through Young Living. We have truly experienced "Wellness, Purpose and Abundance".

Lara Bardizbanian
Star, New York

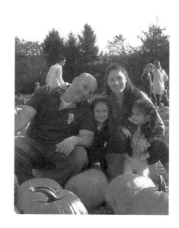

Young Living member since? 2014

Age: 38

Hobbies: Taking care of my kids, my husband, my family and my home, sharing oils, doing voiceovers for radio and TV commercials, volunteering for the kid's theatre company.

Favorite Young Living product? Thieves oil and Household Cleaner

Favorite Young Living product to gift? Frankincense

Favorite Young Living farm or event? The Grand Convention

Describe your day using Young Living products:

Morning: I diffuse oils in the kids' room to help wake them up. Once they're up and dressed, I apply oils down their spine. We have a tea party with tea-cups of NingXia in water. I fill up my water bottle with a few drops of Lemon, Peppermint or some combination depending on what's to come! I alternate between NingXia Red and NingXia Nitro every day around 11 AM when I need a boost.

Afternoon: I use Thieves cleaner to wipe down most everything in my home. I like to experiment with something new every week. This week, I'm using a few drops of Geranium on my skin in the morning and it feels great! Next week—Young Living deodorant!! I spray homemade hand sanitizer on my little one since she sucks her thumb. When either of my kids scrape a knee or elbow, we use Lavender essential oil. In the summer, I have my handy Purification spray bottle ready for action outside!

Evening: At night, we diffuse Lavender in the girl's room to help them have a restful sleep. I put oils on feet during the winter months. And Breathe Again!

What does Young Living mean to you? A few years ago, I prayed to find out what my purpose in life was. I felt like the answer is in nature. I didn't realize what that meant or how it applied to my future. But now, I see how essential oils have helped those I love, how Young Living takes so much care in producing unique products and how I can help make change and share with people that there are options. I'm excited to be part of the Young Living family and anxiously look forward to helping growing.

Lauren Bretz
Diamond, Indiana

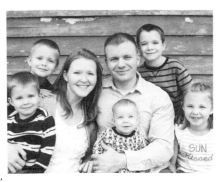

Young Living member since? March 2013
Spouse: Nat Bretz
Age: 31
Hobbies: As a wife and mom of 5 children, hobbies aren't a huge priority. We love clean eating, finding fun new places to eat, traveling, hiking/playing outside and occasionally watching quality movies.

Favorite Young Living product? Frankincense, Juva Spice & Balance Complete
Describe your day using Young Living products:

Morning: I will put Lemon in water before anything else. I will apply Valor to the back of my neck, Peace & Calming over my heart, Frankincense to my forehead, Progessence Plus to my forearms, and Joy on my wrists. Oftentimes, I'll make a cup of tea with Cinnamon Bark, Orange or Cardamom and Young Living Stevia Extract. Supplements: Essentialzyme, Life 5, True Source, Super B, Thyromin, Sulfurzyme and Super C. I will sprinkle JuvaSpice on our eggs and take a shot of NingXia Red! I feel so pampered while I use my Young Living Lavender shampoo and conditioner! My hair has NEVER been better (and I was "poo free" for 5 years!). Lots of bath products!

Afternoon: A smoothie with Balance Complete! Nitro into a shot glass, fill the rest with NingXia Red and add a few drops of essential oils, like Cistus, Orange or Lime. Later, I will use NingXia Red, Nitro, Mineral Essence, Lime and Young Living Stevia Extract. It's so energizing! We use Thieves hand soap and hand purifier, Stress Away roll on and Thieves Spray through the day. I apply Gratitude to mine and my children's wrists and we pray together to stay focused on our need for the Lord and to be thankful.

Evening: I often use a drop of Basil, Thyme, Oregano, Rosemary, Taste of Italy, Lemon or Lime essential oils, depending on what I'm making. I love to clean my kitchen with Thieves Household Cleaner! At night, the children use oils on their feet and Cedarwood on their necks. I use a ton of oils before bed!

What does Young Living mean to you? Young Living truly means wellness, purpose, abundance and community. Young Living means integrity, quality, transparency, and genuine care for others. God has used Young Living to change our lives and we are so thankful. I had no idea when I purchased my starter kit that it would be the gateway into a whole new world of wonder.

Laurie Azzarella
Diamond, Texas

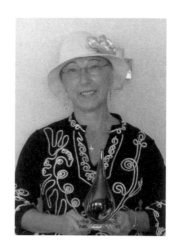

Young Living member since? 1998
Age: 62
Hobbies: Gardening, cooking, teaching
Favorite Young Living product?
Idaho Balsam Fir
Favorite Young Living product to gift?
Deep Relief Roll On
Favorite Young Living farm or event?
Love the Ecuador Farm & Clinic

Describe your day using Young Living products:

Morning: Lemon oil in water, smoothie with Power Meal, JuvaPower, NingXia Red, MindWise and oil of choice. I also take Sulfurzyme, Super B & C, Essentialzyme and capsules of Idaho Blue Spruce, SclarEssence, Lemon, Peppermint, Copaiba and whatever else! I will fill and start using my diffusers! I apply Joy or Shutran oil topically to smell pretty. I will use Lavender soap, Orange Blossom face-wash, ART Moisturizer or Sheerlumé as well as Frankincense. I also use Meadow Mint deodorant, Thieves Dentarome toothpaste and Thieves mouthwash.

Afternoon: I use oils in my massage and reflexology practice along with the AromaDome, so I get lots of aromatherapy during the day!

Evening: I love my bath with oils at night and I will take my supplements at night as well Sulfurzyme, Life 5, OmegaGize and Super Cal. I apply Cel-Lite massage oil to my tummy and thighs. I rub my head with Cedarwood. I diffuse Balsam Fir but also put two drops on my pillow.

When Traveling: Thieves spray, Peppermint, Deep Relief, and DiGize travel in my purse along with samples and business cards. Peace & Calming comes in handy when there's a fussy baby aboard. I also carry NingXia Red packs and Nitro and Slique bars. I also take a diffuser and a bunch of oils in my suitcase.

What does Young Living mean to you? Young Living means HOPE to me: Helping Other People Evolve, as well as empowering them and myself. I am so grateful to God and Gary and Mary for the opportunity they have given to me and to so many others. We all can give hope to this world one person and one oil at a time.

What is your favorite clean eating meal? Raw zucchini spaghetti with marinara and pesto sauce.

Leah Prewitt
Silver, Missouri

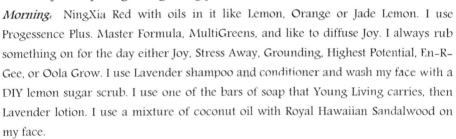

Young Living member since? March 2014

Spouse: Steven Prewitt

Age: 28

Hobbies: Cooking, teaching about health & wellness, being with my family, camping

Favorite Young Living product?

NingXia Red

Favorite Young Living farm or event?

Mona, Utah farm for the Silver Retreat

Describe your day using Young Living products:

Morning: NingXia Red with oils in it like Lemon, Orange or Jade Lemon. I use Progessence Plus. Master Formula, MultiGreens, and like to diffuse Joy. I always rub something on for the day either Joy, Stress Away, Grounding, Highest Potential, En-R-Gee, or Oola Grow. I use Lavender shampoo and conditioner and wash my face with a DIY lemon sugar scrub. I use one of the bars of soap that Young Living carries, then Lavender lotion. I use a mixture of coconut oil with Royal Hawaiian Sandalwood on my face.

Afternoon: More oils rubbed on if the day is going crazy or I need a boost. I sometimes take a capsule of different oils. Right now I'm nursing, so sometimes I will take Fennel.

Evening: After dinner I take one Life 5. In the winter, I rub several oils on the bottoms of my feet.

When Traveling: I try to do all the above. Usually I up my NingXia intake to 4 ounces. I sometimes add in a NingXia Nitro. I take an Inner Defense capsule everyday while on the go. I take a diffuser with us to cleanse the air in hotel rooms. I also use the Thieves Spray on EVERYTHING! Great for airplane seats or shopping carts!

What does Young Living mean to you? It's like loving someone so much and knowing that they have your best interest at heart all the time. When we joined Young Living, we knew that we wanted a safer, healthier option for our family. Our family is top priority on this earth. God provided all we need on this earth and we are so blessed by that! Young Living never settles for less than the best and they bless us with the chance to bless other families.

What is your favorite clean eating meal? Burgers from our beef and homemade buns, with fresh garden veggies and feta cheese. Also fresh fruit like peaches or cantaloupe.

Leanne Peace
Senior Star, Florida

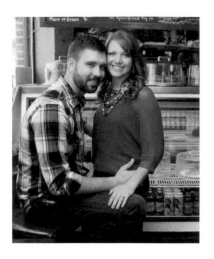

Young Living member since? August 2014

Spouse: Jonny Peace

Age: 28

Hobbies: Reading

Favorite Young Living product?
Lavender and Purification

Favorite Young Living product to gift?
Thieves hand soap

Describe your day using Young Living products:

Morning: I will use Young Living's shampoo and conditioner and Satin Mint Facial Scrub (I break out if I delineate from Young Living products for my face). I drink an ounce of NingXia Red in water every day. When I was dealing with grief through our miscarriage, I would put Joy over my heart each morning before I'd get dressed. Then in rebuilding my body after loss, I'd mix my capsules of Grapefruit and Peppermint oils for the day! My husband will use any mixture of Young Living oils with coconut oil to fix his hair each morning. His barber says it is the healthiest it has ever been!

Afternoon: This ranges from using Thieves hand soap daily or diffusing to applying my favorite Young Living lip balm: Grapefruit! In the summer, I'll also apply our homemade lotion before a trip to the pool and add a few drops of Purification oil to the laundry when doing chores!

Evening: I always use Thieves cleaner mixed with water to clean up after dinner! My nighttime routine also consists of using Thieves toothpaste, rubbing on Ledum and Citrus Fresh on my thighs and belly, and diffusing Lavender to encourage rest.

When Traveling: I never EVER leave without Lavender & Peppermint! I will use Lavender after being in the sun and Peppermint to help during the flights.

What does Young Living mean to you? Young Living means positive change, motivation, health, wellness, encouragement, setting and meeting goals, building relationships, working together and endless opportunity! It has only brought good things into our lives!

What is your favorite clean eating meal? Any seafood (shrimp and salmon are our easiest and favorites), sweet potatoes and veggies!

Les Wright
Crown Diamond, Alabama

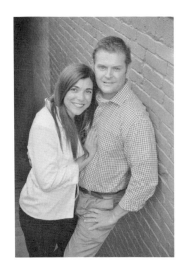

Young Living member since? September 2012
Spouse: Kelli Wright
Age: 45
Hobbies: Hunting, outdoor stuff, running, keeping up with the kids
Favorite Young Living product?
Frankincense

Favorite Young Living farm or event? The Mona, Utah Farm

Describe your day using Young Living products:

Morning: Two ounces of NingXia Red with Lemon and Peppermint dropped in. An hour after breakfast I use Sulfurzyme and then one hour after lunch 2 more Sulfurzyme. During the day: 1 capsule of Idaho Blue Spruce, Golden Rod, Copaiba; 3 drops each. Peppermint before exercising.

Evening: Two ounces of NingXia Red and also Life 5 before bed. I use Young Living's toothpaste and shampoo.

What does Young Living mean to you? Young Living oils and oil-infused products have revolutionized our family's wellness plan. We use them every day.

What is your favorite clean eating meal? Chicken thighs on the grill.

Lindsay Haymes

Gold, Missouri

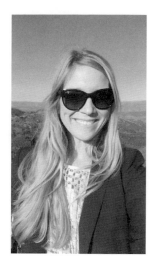

Young Living member since? July 2013

Age: 31

Hobbies: Traveling, being with family and friends, lake activities, hosting parties and events.

Favorite Young Living product?
Peppermint

Favorite Young Living farm or event? Mona, Utah Draft Horse Festival

Describe your day using Young Living products:

Morning: I start my day with a cocktail of Essentialzyme, JuvaTone, Longevity, ImmuPro and Super C tablets washed down with NingXia Red. As for my getting ready routine, I use Progessence Plus on my wrists, DIY Tea Tree face scrub, Thieves toothpaste, Young Living deodorant and Genesis lotion. Truly, there's not a product I use in the morning that's not Young Living!

Afternoon: Right now I'm using Faith and Believe oils on my chest and Valor or Valor II on the back of my neck in the afternoons for a boost! I am also in love with Light the Fire oil launched at the 2015 Convention!

Evening: Before bed I use Cedarwood and apply oils to my feet for immune system support. In my home I am often diffusing Christmas Spirit and Lemon Myrtle or whatever other combination I feel like!

What does Young Living mean to you? Young Living has made me a more conscientious consumer. I'm obsessed with ingredients and avoiding toxic chemicals in our environment now like never before. I love that I don't HAVE to spend time researching what products to buy for my home and personal care, because I trust Young Living's all natural and quality standards completely! I am so grateful to Gary Young and Young Living for the years I am adding on to my life because of the level of health and wellness I have achieved with Young Living, which I will continue to enjoy for the rest of my life!

Lindsey Gremont
Crown Diamond, Texas

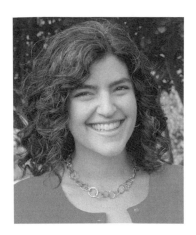

Young Living member since? July 2013
Spouse: Evan Gremont
Age: 37
Hobbies: Cooking, hiking, reading, DIY
Favorite Young Living product? Detoxzyme
Favorite Young Living farm or event?
Highland Flats Winter Harvest!

Describe your day using Young Living products:

Morning: A shot of NingXia Red with Tangerine and Frankincense. Digest + Cleanse, Detoxzyme, Sulfurzyme, a capsule with SclarEssence, Longevity. Super C. Then 'Happy Protocol': Joy, Harmony, Valor & White Angelica. AromaBright toothpaste. I use my own DIY shampoo and conditioner with Rosemary oil. I make my own DIY shower gel with Ylang Ylang and Idaho Blue Spruce oils. I also use DIY deodorant with Petitgrain and other oils. DIY hair styling product with Lavender, Rosemary, Cedarwood. I also use the ART moisturizer, Orange Blossom face wash and diffuse Joy and Lemon!

Afternoon: Another shot of NingXia Red. I take Essentialzymes-4 with meals. I diffuse what I need to focus – usually Rosemary, Jade Lemon or Clarity. I'll also use my DIY foaming hand soap.

Evening: I diffuse some Peace & Calming and Lavender to unwind. Love to add oils to our baths with Epsom salt. My daughter gets to pick which ones she wants! I take a Digest + Cleanse and a Detoxzyme before bed 3-4 times a week. On the days when I don't take those, I take a few Life 5's before bed. I also use Valor and Cedarwood and some immune support oils. My favorites: Thieves, Ginger, Lemongrass and Ravintsara.

When Traveling: I usually take about 30 oils with me when I travel! Same routine!

What does Young Living mean to you? Young Living to me means integrity and wellness. I advocate knowing my farmer and I love that we get to really know how exactly Young Living grows and distills our oils. Young Living is much more than essential oils, it is about living a vibrantly healthy life. We have to load our bodies with nutrients, get rid of toxins and manage our stress to be truly WELL. I am so blessed to teach everyone how to do the same!

What is your favorite clean eating meal? As a real food blogger, I am all about eating completely unprocessed REAL food. We follow a Weston A. Price style (WAPF) diet.

Lori Gasca

Diamond, Texas

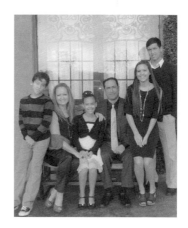

Young Living member since? 2009
Spouse: Michael Gasca
Age: 45
Hobbies: Faux painting, salvaging old things and making them new, chasing our kiddos
Favorite Young Living product? ImmuPro
Favorite Young Living farm or event?
As of now, Young Living convention, but I have a feeling it will be the Diamond Retreat.

Describe your day using Young Living products:

Morning: We start our morning off with a delicious drink of 1-2 ounces of NingXia Red, a capful of Braggs ACV, 2-3 drops of a citrus oil (usually Lemon or Lime) over crushed ice and about 10 ounces of water! If I feel the need for a little more energy, I will add a NingXia Nitro too. So delicious and nutritious. Gets the plumbing going first thing in the morning! A great way to start the day! As for applying oils...it just depends on what I need. I have been working my way through the Freedom Sleep and Freedom Release kits with AMAZING results! I like to focus on one of the kits offered because it gives me a good routine to follow...Reconnect, Feelings, etc. We also kick start the day with Super C chewables. Finally, Thieves toothpaste!

Afternoon: Depending on how the day is going, I might need a Nitro for that boost of energy. During the day, I have also taken my Life 5 and Essentialzyme! The diffuser is often running most of the day in some part of the home as well. I clean all day long with Thieves household cleaner! I also use a DIY non-toxic air purifier with oils!

Evening: I love ending my day with an oily Epsom bath. We take the majority of our supplements at night. OmegaGize, Sulfurzyme, Master Formula, PD 80/20, Super B, JuvaTone, Inner Defense, Digest + Cleanse. We get a beautiful night's sleep and boost the immune system at the same time with ImmuPro!

What does Young Living mean to you? Life change. Freedom. Health. Happiness. Empowerment. I have a college degree, have held professional jobs and had many entrepreneurial businesses. None of them come close to the pure joy Young Living gives me. I truly have the power to change my future and the lives of those I adore on this earth! And so do you! Today is your day...Make it happen!

Marcella Vonn Harting, PhD

Royal Crown Diamond, Arizona

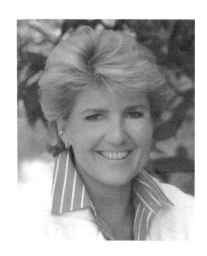

Young Living member since? 1992

Spouse: Jim Harting

Hobbies: Water or snow skiing, hiking, golf, tennis, reading

Favorite Young Living product?
Sacred Mountain oil

Favorite Young Living farm or event?
St. Maries Farm and the Grand Convention

Describe your day using Young Living products:

Morning: Morning Start or Sensation bath gel in the shower then Orange Blossom for face. Geranium oil as deodorant or Young Living deodorant. Sheerlumé and Creme Masque for face. Thieves toothpaste and mouthwash for oral hygiene and Sacred Mountain oil on chest for protection and grounding throughout my day. I use oils on my feet daily. Some mornings I take a Power Meal shake. I will also take 5-8 enzymes on empty stomach before breakfast, 2-4 oz. NingXia Red and MindWise with breakfast. Also, Master Formula and Super C.

Afternoon: Enzymes

Evening: Enzymes and Life 5

When Traveling: I will take capsules of 10-12 drops of Clove oil. Enzymes, vitamin C, NingXia Red and Nitro

What does Young Living mean to you? Young Living is an integral part of the Harting family. I've been involved with this company 24 years; it is who we are. My son, Dallas is a Diamond and my daughter, Kortni is a Platinum, (husband Luke is a Silver). We work full time traveling and supporting our organizations. I was a stay at home mom and Young Living became my career, my purpose and my PASSION. The products are life changing—physically, emotionally and financially. I have grown into a leader for my organization, a writer, and speaker and have even gone back to school to receive a dual PhD in Psychoneurology and Integrative Health & Thriving.

What is your favorite clean eating meal? Lean and green (Grass feed steak and salad).

Mary Starr Carter

Diamond, Florida

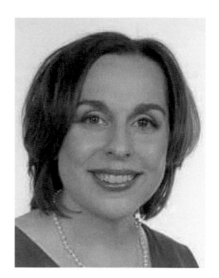

Young Living member since? 1999
Spouse: Jay Carter
Age: 40
Hobbies: Tennis, healthy cooking, writing
Favorite Young Living product? Life 5
Favorite Young Living product to gift?
ART Beauty Serum
Favorite Young Living farm or event?
The France Farm

Describe your day using Young Living products:

Morning: First thing is Cedarwood, then later Thyromin, Pure Protein Complete, Super B, 2 ounces of NingXia Red and Mineral Essence. Progessence Plus and EndoFlex on my neck, Frankincense on my chest, Joy over my heart, Cel-Lite massage oil on my belly and legs. I love Orange Blossom Facial Wash and the ART Renewal Serum and moisturizer. My favorite shampoo and conditioner is the Lavender Mint.
Afternoon: Essentialzyme, Super B, Sulfurzyme, NingXia Red with Mineral Essence. I inhale Peppermint and Joy. If I'm working I might diffuse Motivation, Abundance or Joy. I love any of the citrus oils or Peppermint in my water throughout the day. We use all the Thieves household cleaning products.
Evening: Essentialzyme, Sulfurzyme, BLM, Life 5, relax while diffusing Shutran. I use Lavender and Cedarwood before bed.

What does Young Living mean to you? One word: Freedom. It's given me freedom to leave my Chiropractic practice, homeschool my kids, and it allowed my husband to release his 80 hour work week in corporate America. We've been able to hire help around the house so we can do what we love without sacrificing family time. My husband and I are now healthier and happier than we've ever been because of Young Living. The lifestyle they inspire us to live, the products they give us, and the income all are helping us reach our highest potential and help others do the same.

Megan Jobes
Silver, Missouri

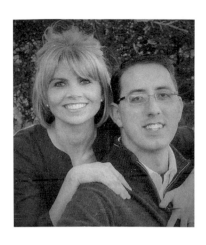

Young Living member since? 2014

Spouse: Tucker Jobes

Age: 31

Hobbies: Running and training for my first marathon

Favorite Young Living product?
Lavender Hand & Body Lotion

Favorite Young Living product to gift?
Peppermint or Thieves Cleaner

Favorite Young Living farm or event? I'm so excited I got to attend the Silver Retreat in Mona, Utah! It was amazing!

Describe your day using Young Living products:

Morning: I do the oil-cleansing method using Tea Tree & Elemi and almond oil on my face. Citrus Fresh. Purification with grape seed oil as deodorant, I'll apply a drop of Joy over my heart or White Angelica on my shoulders or back of neck. A couple of times a week, I eat Einkorn pancakes. I will also take Master Formula, NingXia and diffuse a combination of Joy & Citrus Fresh. I use Thieves AromaBright toothpaste with a drop of Orange. Capsule every day of Thieves, Orange, DiGize, Thyme, or Spearmint. On my hair I put Peace & Calming to tame fly-aways.

Afternoon: I will drink water with couple drops Citrus Fresh. With 2 young kids, Nitro is a necessity. My daughter gets a drop of a citrus oil in applesauce. I clean little messes with Thieves cleaner. I use wool dryer balls with Stress Away in the dryer.

Evening: KidScents shampoo for my kids as well as myself. I use Lavender conditioner for my hair and to shave and then Peppermint-Cedarwood Soap and Lavender lotion! Thieves toothpaste (my kids brush with this, too), and Thieves floss. I do the oil-cleansing method again with Elemi, Mel-A and almond oil and use Young Living lip balm before bed. I have a couple oils open on my nightstand, but my favorite is Lavender. For the kids, we will put oils on their feet and spray Cedarwood in their rooms.

What does Young Living mean to you? What Young Living means to me is empowerment. As a wife and a mommy, I am able to take on my family's health with the use of Young Living in a natural and toxic-free direction. The feeling of being completely confident in every single product we use is invaluable. I also feel blessed that I get to lead other families to this path as well.

Melissa Koehler

Royal Crown Diamond, California

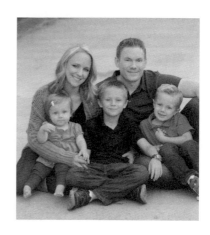

Young Living member since? June 2013

Spouse: Mark Koehler

Age: 35

Hobbies: Photography, crafts, dreaming up ways to organize my home

Favorite Young Living product? Thieves

Favorite Young Living product to gift? Thieves

Favorite Young Living farm or event?
I loved the Ecuador farm!

Describe your day using Young Living products:

Morning: In the mornings, I love to use Thieves and Peppermint. I like to diffuse different oils in my office. I use Valor and put Motivation behind my ears.

Afternoon: I apply Peppermint on my wrists and use Valor and NingXia.

Evening: Stress Away, Orange Blossom face wash, Mint scrub, Boswellia cream and Wolfberry eye cream. Peace & Calming on my feet. I use Frankincense and a blend of Citrus Fresh and Ledum before bed. I will also take a capsule of Grapefruit.

When Traveling: I have a whole case of oils I keep with me but some most used ones are Thieves and Cedarwood. I also take NingXia.

What does Young Living mean to you? Young Living means that I can help my family lead a healthy lifestyle. My children can feel confident knowing that we are promoting our family's wellness with essential oils and good food. Young Living has brought so much freedom and confidence to my life.

Melissa Poepping
Crown Diamond, Minnesota

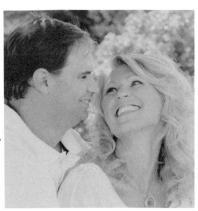

Young Living member since? 2000

Spouse: Wayne Poepping

Age: 36

Hobbies: Gardening, swimming, muscle cars, recreational shooting

Favorite Young Living product?
Sulfurzyme

Favorite Young Living farm or event?
Beauty School

Describe your day using Young Living products:

Morning: Thieves toothpaste, the Young Living skincare line (yes, all of it). Progessence Plus, NingXia Red, Nitro, MindWise, Sulfurzyme.

Afternoon: Harmony over my solar plexus, Joy over my heart, Valor on my wrists and White Angelica swept down my arms. And more NingXia Red!

Evening: Shutran and more Sulfurzyme.

What does Young Living mean to you? The health benefits we as a family are experiencing with Young Living have been PHENOMENAL and I always feel obligated to share this resource with others. As it turns out, living a healthy lifestyle is craved in most communities! In no time at all, we've created a movement that quickly caught on! Showing others how to create a Young Living lifestyle impacts generations to come and allows people to take charge of their wellness by creating their own health care system and, if they so choose, their own economy!

What is your favorite clean eating meal? We eat pretty good so my favorite is when we do 100 Mile Meals.

Michelle Johnson
Silver, Missouri

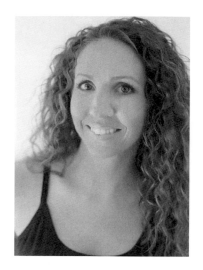

Young Living member since? 2012

Spouse: Brad Johnson

Age: 33

Hobbies: Cooking, teaching the kids church, everything creative: painting, murals, house projects, crafts with kids, outdoor adventures

Favorite Young Living product?

Lavender lotion

Favorite Young Living farm or event?

The farm in Idaho for Silver Retreat

Describe your day using Young Living products:

Morning: Master Formula vitamins. I drink NingXia Red at breakfast... I cleanse my face with a DIY-made sugar scrub that contains a citrus oil and Geranium. I mix Frankincense in coconut oil as a facial moisturizer. I love AromaBright toothpaste. I apply oils to my Oil Armed diffuser bracelet. My favorite combos are: a citrus oil with Idaho Balsam Fir or Believe. I use Thieves cleaner on the kitchen counters.

Afternoon: After my shower, which let's be honest, often doesn't happen until afternoon time….I use Lavender lotion. I often diffuse oils of all sorts. Some of my favorites are Purification, Christmas Spirit and Idaho Blue Spruce and citrus oils. I usually go to my oil bag and choose what oil I feel like for that day. I really love to wear Idaho Blue Spruce, Sandalwood, Patchouli, Idaho Balsam Fir, Tangerine, Inner Child, Trauma Life and Believe. I also from time to time take a capsule with Fennel oil.

Evening: Evenings are a bath time for baby. I use one drop of Lavender and one drop of Gentle Babies in the bath water along with KidsScents body wash. After the bath, I massage my baby with coconut oil and one drop of Lavender. Heavenly! In the diffuser in the evenings you will find: Cedarwood & Lavender or Myrtle.

What does Young Living mean to you? Young Living, summed up into one word: Comfort. I live each day trying to provide the happiest and healthiest life for myself and my family. It brings me such comfort to know that beyond healthy eating and exercise, Young Living has us covered head to toe. From the skin care we put on our bodies, to the supplements we put in our bodies, to the products we use around us... I find comfort in knowing that I am using high quality, natural products that come from a company with such high integrity!

Myra Yarbrough
Crown Diamond, Alabama

Young Living member since? 2012
Spouse: Ernie Yarbrough
Age: 33
Hobbies: Blogging, decorating, cooking
Favorite Young Living product?
Thieves
Favorite Young Living farm or event?
St. Maries Lavender Farm

Describe your day using Young Living products:

Morning: In the morning I love to drink my NingXia Red with Orange oil – yum! I get all my diffusers going with citrus oils and a mint oil. The crisp citrus aroma is very uplifting. I apply EndoFlex to my neck and mid-back, then inhale deeply from my hands. Valor always goes on my wrists and Joy over my heart. I brush my teeth with Thieves AromaBright and take care of my face with the ART skin care system. Love that stuff! I use the Satin Mint Scrub 2-3 times a week. If I don't have time to fix a meal, I will have a Pure Protein shake for breakfast after I work out. I'm a fanatic about having my counters clean, so I usually do a quick wipe down with my beloved Thieves Household Cleaner.

Afternoon: I usually refill the diffusers, apply En-R-Gee to my wrists and sit down to work while my 3 year old naps.

Evening: Refill bedroom diffusers: Lavender and Cedarwood (LOVE that!). I use my Thieves AromaBright toothpaste and the ART line. I apply Sheerlumé to my face (totally addicted!) then Life 5, Lavender lotion with Gentle Baby oil all over my growing belly.

What does Young Living mean to you? Unlike so many who have had life changing results from using the oils and the oil infused products, our experience has been a little different. Young Living just fits perfectly into what we were already doing for our health and wellness. I am so grateful to feel empowered to care for my family in our day-to-day life. I love that I don't have to worry about the products that my kids are exposed to – they are safe and that's a huge blessing.

What is your favorite clean eating meal? I love scrambled eggs topped with sautéed vegetables and with some nitrate free bacon on the side.

Nancy Orlen Weber

Diamond, New Jersey

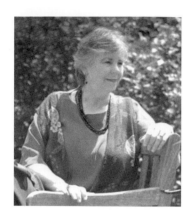

Young Living member since? 2003
Spouse: Dick Weber
Age: 71
Hobbies: Writing, dancing, drawing, traveling, music, petting squirrels, groundhogs and deer
Favorite Young Living product?
Highest Potential oil
Favorite Young Living product to gift?
Abundance oil

Favorite Young Living farm or event? Grand Convention, especially when it's in Utah
Describe your day using Young Living products:

Morning: Morning Start Bath Gel, Lavender shampoo, ART Gentle Cleanser followed by Satin Facial Scrub Mint. For my face: Rose, Frankincense then the Renewal Serum and Sheerlumé. For anointing and prayer time I use Release, Gathering, Endoflex, Magnify Your Purpose, Highest Potential, Brain Power, Awaken, Sacred Frankincense, Frankincense, Palo Santo, Cedarwood, Balsam Fir, Harmony or Abundance. I use the following supplements: BLM, Sulfurzyme, NingXia Red, NingXia Nitro, True Source, Life 5, OmegaGize, Longevity and Inner Defense. Essentialzyme, Essentialzymes-4, and Allerzyme.

Afternoon: In the afternoon I diffuse a citrus oil, Clarity or Christmas Spirit. I will apply Helichrysum, Juniper, Highest Potential and Abundance before eating. I also often take Inner Defense, BLM, Sulfurzyme, NingXia Nitro. Essentialzyme, Essentialzymes-4, and Allerzyme.

Evening: I like to diffuse Lavender or Balsam Fir. Inner Defense, BLM, Sulfurzyme, NingXia Nitro, OmegaGize. Essentialzyme, Essentialzymes-4, and Allerzyme. Topically, I use Cypress, Blue Cypress, Balsam Fir, RutaVaLa. Late evening: Life 5.

What does Young Living mean to you? Young Living's mission is my mission. Since childhood my passion is to make a difference, to leave this earth knowing I have helped this planet and all who live here. Young Living fulfills my passion and offers me the incredible blessing of authentically seeking wellness, purpose and abundance.

Nathan Petty
Crown Diamond, California

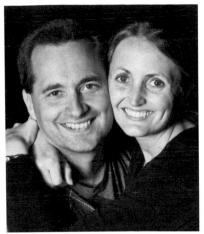

Young Living member since? October 2013

Spouse: Jessica Petty

Age: 40

Hobbies: Surfing, photography, drums, videography, travel and family time.

Favorite Young Living product?
Thieves

Favorite Young Living product to gift?
Lemon

Favorite Young Living farm or event? Global Leadership Mediterranean Cruise 2015

Describe your day using Young Living products:

Morning: Thieves toothpaste, Thieves oil, OolaFun, Lemon, Citrus Fresh.

Afternoon: Frankincense and whatever else grabs my attention.

Evening: Thieves toothpaste, Valor, Lavender bath gel, Peppermint.

When Traveling: All of the above. No real routine other than Thieves and Frankincense and whatever else I'm feeling that day.

What does Young Living mean to you? It is very fulfilling to share natural products, freedom of time and means, friendships, travel, time to help others, entrepreneurship, developing talents.

What is your favorite clean eating meal? Don't ask such hard questions! Veggie pizza is always tasty.

Pam Edwards
Diamond, Canada

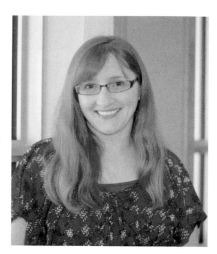

Young Living member since? 2011

Spouse: Gary Edwards

Age: 39

Hobbies: Watching Antique Roadshow, listening to audiobooks when traveling and traveling a lot!

Favorite Young Living product? NingXia Nitro

Favorite Young Living farm or event? The Hawaiian Sandalwood Farm

Describe your day using Young Living products:

Morning: In the mornings, I get my diffuser running. I usually put in Abundance with whatever area of Oola I would like to grow in by choosing one of the Oola oils to go with it. I also take a NingXia Red packet and then around mid-morning grab a Nitro to finish out the morning strong. I also could sip on AlkaLime all day long. There is something about the little bubbles that make me happy. I use the Lavender shampoo and conditioner then pamper my face with the KidScents lotion with Frankincense added.

Afternoon: By 2 PM, I usually try to get in a nap with the little one. In order for my brain to shut down and be quiet, I apply a drop of Vetiver to my wrist. Depending on the day, I will have another NingXia Red packet and Nitro after my nap.

Evening: To unwind, I pull out my Vetiver and sometimes take an Immupro for added immune boosting. The melatonin in it sure helps with a restful night's sleep.

When Traveling: Nitro and DiGize are a must. In 2013 on the Hawaii trip, I had horrible motion sickness on the airplane. I decided to take a Nitro and within minutes all the dizziness and nausea was gone. I now make sure to have Nitro before every flight. I even took 6 boxes of Nitro with us on the 2015 Global Leadership Cruise. We went through 5 of the boxes. Works great for bus rides up to the farms as well.

What does Young Living mean to you? Young Living Essential Oils first changed the way we looked at our health. For two years we used the oils in our home, but not with the consistency we do now. Then in August 2013, I found out there was a business side. I knew I had to share with my friends and family. I went from a single 19 year old mom of one child on welfare to a married woman with 8 children now being able to provide for all our family's needs. It feels amazing to be wealthy in so many areas thanks to Young Living. Wealthy in health, friendships, business, and finances.

Patricia Gwee
Crown Diamond, Singapore

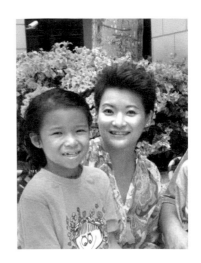

Young Living member since? October 2010

Spouse: P-Wa Tang

Age: 47

Hobbies: Listening to music, arts & culture, learning about natural therapies, spirituality, meditation, reading, Zentangle

Favorite Young Living product?

I love Peppermint

Favorite Young Living product to gift?

Gratitude oil

Favorite Young Living farm or event? International Grand Convention

Describe your day using Young Living products:

Morning: Sacred Frankincense, Believe, Highest Potential, Progessence Phyto Plus. Supplements: Power Meal, NingXia Red, Sulfurzyme, OmegaGize, Super C, Multi-Greens, Essentialzymes-4, Mineral Essence, MindWise.

Afternoon: NingXia Red, Nitro, same supplements as morning except no MindWise.

Evening: Same supplements as afternoon and Detoxzyme.

When Traveling: Lots of Ning Xia Red & Nitro plus the supplements that I usually take.

What does Young Living mean to you? Young Living has enabled me to live my dream! Being involved with Young Living has not only provided me with the tools and ability to be a catalyst to improve the health and wellness of the precious people around me, but it has also gifted me with deep lasting, personal life lessons: independ- ence, self-empowerment, and self-care. I have grown to learn that it's through truly knowing oneself that you can reach out to others in a genuine and authentic way. Being of service to others is one of life's greatest gifts. It is through inspiring others to care that I have attained great fulfillment. I am humbled and grateful to Young Living which has indeed provided me with better Wellness, a Purpose in life and an Abun- dant life, with which I can carry on blessing more and more people.

Rachel Holland
Diamond, Texas

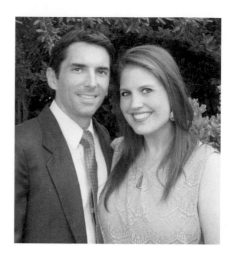

Young Living member since? 2013
Spouse: Ryan Holland
Age: 35
Hobbies: Homeschooling, playing piano, blogging
Favorite Young Living product? NingXia
Favorite Young Living farm or event?
St. Maries Lavender Farm

Describe your day using Young Living products:

Morning: Immediately after waking up I take Young Living's ComforTone supplement. I use Morning Start Bath Gel and Copaiba shampoo & conditioner and put on a layer of ART Light Moisturizer. Before breakfast I drink NingXia Red with Orange added. I take Essentialzymes-4 with breakfast. I clean the kitchen using Young Living Thieves cleaner concentrate. During homeschool time I diffuse Brian Power or other favorite oils. Everyone gets a chewable Super C!

Afternoon: For lunch I drink a Balance Complete shake. I usually drink a Ningxia Nitro around 2:00 and apply En-R-Gee topically if needed. During the late afternoon I diffuse Christmas Spirit and a citrus oil (even in the summer)!

Evening: I love incorporating essential oils into our dinner! Black Pepper and Oregano are two of my favorites to incorporate into recipes. I typically take another Essentialzymes-4 again with my evening meal. After dinner, it's time for baths for the kids with Young Living KidScents Shampoo and Bath Gel. Dream Catcher in the diffuser for the boys' room, RC for the girls' room, Peace & Calming in the master bedroom. I love ART cleanser and toner then Sandalwood lotion. Cinnamon Lip Balm.

What does Young Living mean to you? Young Living has blessed our family in so many ways, but one way that I'm able to share about is that Young Living products have given me back the energy I need for daily life with 4 children. We have incorporated Young Living products everywhere possible in our home and knowing that I'm providing our family with toxin-free products that also help to promote healthy bodies is invaluable!

What is your favorite clean eating meal? Spaghetti made with fresh ingredients!

Rebecca Ishum
Gold, Missouri

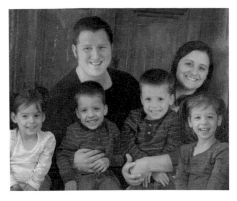

Young Living member since? 2014
Spouse: Sean Ishum
Age: 30
Hobbies: Does raising quadruplets count? Because that is my main activity. That and Young Living and writing on my blog.

Favorite Young Living product? Wolfberry Eye Cream
Favorite Young Living product to gift? Friends: Peace & Calming, Teachers: Thieves

Describe your day using Young Living products:

Morning: I use Morning Start bar soap, Copaiba shampoo and conditioner, and Orange Blossom Face Wash in the shower. Then I use Mountain Mist deodorant, ART Toner, Wolfberry Eye Cream, and Sheerlumé as I'm getting ready for the day. I also use Stress Away, Valor and Joy to help myself get my mood in order. Ningxia Red happens when I hit the kitchen. After breakfast, I use Thieves AromaBright toothpaste.

Afternoon: I use Thieves Cleaner for messes and spills and Thieves Hand Soap.

Evening: I wash my face with ART Face Wash, then ART Toner, then Wolfberry Eye Cream and Sheerlumé. Teeth are brushed with Thieves AromaBright toothpaste. I put something soothing in the diffuser like Lavender to promote sleep and use Forgiveness, Inner Child and Grounding topically.

When Traveling: When we are traveling, I take Inner Defense daily, double my Ningxia Red intake, pack Thieves Wipes and Thieves Hand Sanitizer and use Frankincense over my lungs. I also use my little travel Orb diffuser with Thieves to keep my immune system up.

What does Young Living mean to you? With preemie quadruplets, we look for anything that will boost our immune systems. Young Living helped our family find that new level of wellness! Our new lifestyle is not only easy to incorporate into our family, but we have found that our kids absolutely love their oils as well. On the other side, the business has been a huge financial blessing to our family! I guess the best way to say it is that Young Living has been life changing on every level!

What is your favorite clean eating meal? We really love Greek food! Shawarma Chicken marinated in oil and spices, topped with tzatziki sauce, and a cucumber, tomato salad on the side. So yummy and full of flavor!

Rob Rinato
Diamond, Florida

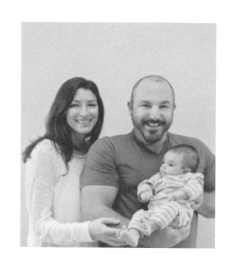

YL member since? 2009

Age: 33

Hobbies: Travel, beach days, boating, playing with our son, collecting Young Living oils

Favorite Young Living product? Valor

Favorite Product to Gift? Everyday Oils

Favorite Young Living farm or event? Master Leader Retreat in Ecuador

Describe your day using Young Living products:

Morning: Diffuse Citrus Fresh + Abundance, NingXia Red, MultiGreens, Enzymes, Sulfurzyme, Thieves toothpaste, Lavender shampoo, Morning Start bath gel, apply Shutran and have a fruit smoothie with Balance Complete.

Afternoon: Diffuse tangerine and Frankincense, drink more NingXia Red or Nitro if needed, Lavender for nap time for our son Roman. Peppermint or Clarity if working in the office

Evening: NingXia Red spritzer with dinner (sparkling water with 2 ounces NingXia Red and 2 drops of Grapefruit or Tangerine oils), Lavender and Cedarwood in the diffuser and applied for bedtime, Thieves toothpaste and floss, MultiGreens, Life 5 , enzymes, Sulfurzyme before bed.

When Traveling: DiGize, Peppermint, Lavender, Lemon, Bon Voyage Travel Pack, Thieves hand purifier, NingXia Red and Nitro.

What does Young Living mean to you? In one word, Young Living means *lifestyle* for us. It allows us to build a business based on our values. It has given us the time freedom to be stay at home parents while we work together to help others realize their dreams of Wellness, Purpose and Abundance.

What is your favorite clean eating meal? Grilled shrimp over organic greens with Lemon essential oil, vinaigrette, goat cheese, walnuts, dried cranberries, and clementine slices!

Ryan Prather
Diamond, Colorado

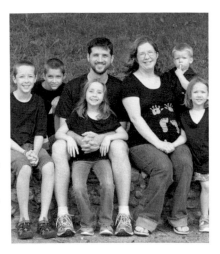

Young Living member since? 2011
Spouse: Kim Prather
Age: 35
Hobbies: Woodworking and computers
Favorite Young Living product? There are so many I like, I don't know if I can choose one.
Favorite Young Living farm or event? Diamond Retreat and the Croatia Farm

Describe your day using Young Living products:

Morning: Sulfurzyme, BLM, MultiGreens (Master Formula or True Source, whichever is available), Super B, Super C, Shutran, Idaho Blue Spruce and two ounces of NingXia Red. We use KidScents shampoo to bathe our little ones.
Afternoon: Thieves household cleaner and other Thieves products to clean everything in the house.
Evening: Sulfurzyme, BLM, MultiGreens, Valor, Peace & Calming
When Traveling: Nothing special right now, although we drank a lot of NingXia Red on the Diamond retreat!

What does Young Living mean to you? Freedom! Young Living has allowed me to quit my job and come home to be with my family full-time! Recently, my wife lost her grandmother and I was able to tell her to just leave and go to be with her family and I stayed home with the kids. Most other 9-to-5 jobs wouldn't allow you to do something like that! Or I would have had to take time off which could have messed up other plans for that time off.

What is your favorite clean eating meal? Steak salad with vinaigrette ing! AMAZING!!!

Sandi Boudreau
Diamond, California

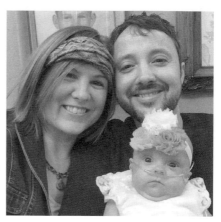

Young Living member since? 2013

Spouse: Kyler Boudreau

Hobbies: Grill, do things with the family, movies, read, coffee with friends, Young Living

Favorite Young Living product? NingXia

Favorite Young Living product to gift? NingXia Red or Nitro

Favorite Young Living farm or event? The Grand Convention, hands down

Describe your day using Young Living products:

Morning: In my morning shower, I use Young Living's Lavender or Copaiba Vanilla shampoo and I love the Orange Blossom Facial Wash. I also take OmegaGize, Multi-Greens, NingXia Red and BLM daily.

Afternoon: NITRO! I also diffuse any of the emotional oils. Current favorites are Grounding, Forgiveness and Acceptance. I also love diffusing any citrus oils! *Evening:* We diffuse in the evenings. We usually diffuse an emotionally grounding oil in the evening. My hubby uses Cedarwood on his head at night. On the bottoms of our feet, we use the oils from the Feelings Kit. I often use Valor throughout the day. *When Traveling:* We take all our oils with us. And I do mean ALL. My Aroma Com- plete is with me right now — on this trip.

What does Young Living mean to you? Young Living is a lifestyle change: supplements, home cleaning products, skin and facial care, and of course the oils that support every body system. Our hope is to share the products with others who aim to take charge of their health. We believe that what we do, think, eat and believe shapes our world. Being well means feeling well, and since the oils also support our emotions—that makes all the difference!

What is your favorite clean eating meal? We love an organic salad with kale, spinach, carrots, coconut slivers, walnuts, cranberries and grilled chicken. We add a homemade dressing made up of olive oil, 4 drops of Lemon oil, balsamic vinegar and red vino. Mmmm!

Sara Wallace
Diamond, Oklahoma

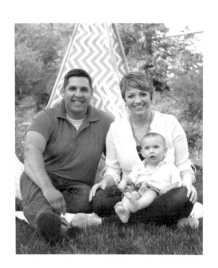

Young Living member since? 2008

Spouse: Justin Wallace

Age: 25

Hobbies: Gardening, water activities, bringing the office to the back patio, guitar

Favorite Young Living product? Everything!

Favorite Young Living product to gift? Massage oils, roll ons, and ClaraDerm for baby showers

Favorite Young Living farm or event? St. Maries Farm

Describe your day using Young Living products:

Morning: Thieves toothpaste and Thieves mouthwash immediately afterwards. Then Lavender Mint shampoo & conditioner, and Valor, Lemon Sandalwood, Thieves, or Peppermint Cedarwood bar soap. ART Gentle Foaming Cleanser, Toner, Renewal Serum and Boswellia Wrinkle Cream. I love L' Brianté lip gloss. We also use Lavender lotion, Sandalwood Moisture Cream, and Animal Scents Ointment – my favorite moisturizing products. Then NingXia and the diffuser combo of the day.

Afternoon: More NingXia Red! Slique Essence in my water bottle, Super C, BLM, Essentialzymes-4 or Detoxzyme. I rotate my supplements throughout the day. Pre gym: Peppermint and Idaho Blue Spruce. Post gym: Cel-Lite Magic or Ortho Sport massage oils. Thieves Spray, Super B, Nutmeg and En-R-Gee.

Evening: Thieves Cleaner to spruce up the house. I wear Abundance & Rose oils. Refill the diffusers. Then if it's class time, the NingXia Red and class oils are sure to be free flowing. Before bed: Thyromin. Lavender… SleepyIze for the little man. We often diffuse Thieves, Raven or RC overnight, especially during the winter months.

What does Young Living mean to you? Young Living, to me, means freedom. It means the freedom to live my life to the fullest. To be well and enjoy wellness in my family. The freedom to pursue adding value to lives of families all over the globe. The freedom to attract and enjoy abundance. And I get excited because I know there are so many more people out there who will be able to experience what I am experiencing by being a part of this incredible company—this incredible community!

Sarah Lee

Diamond, Washington

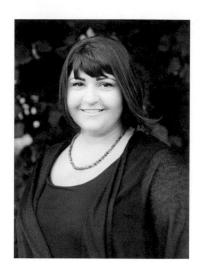

YL member since? May 2013

Spouse: Gary Lee

Age: 39

Hobbies: Crafts, gardening, sewing and entertaining company

Favorite Young Living product? Valor and ImmuPro

Favorite Young Living product to gift: Stress Away Roll On

Favorite Young Living Farm or Event? The Ecuador Farm

Describe your day using Young Living products:

Morning: I use Orange Blossom Facial Wash, Satin Mint Scrub and Morning Start bath gel in the shower every day. I use the Lavender lotion when I get out. On my face goes ART toner, Essential Beauty Serum, Boswellia Wrinkle Cream. I put Joy over my heart when I get out of the shower. I drink a NingXia Red, sometimes with added es- sential oils, sometimes with Perrier mixed in.

Evening: I use many different Young Living oils, supplements and products through-out the day and evening. I am always changing it up depending on the need.

When Traveling: When I travel I always take NingXia Red and ImmuPro with me as well and a couple of bags of essential oils.

What does Young Living mean to you? Young Living is about Wellness, Purpose and Abundance. Young Living is about personal development and growth. It's about work-ing together and helping people. Young Living is about changing people's lives.

What is your favorite clean eating meal? I love a good grilled steak.

Sera Johnson
Crown Diamond, Texas

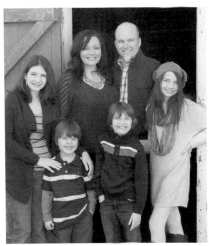

Young Living member since? 2006

Spouse: Darren Johnson

Age: 39

Hobbies: Traveling the world with my family. Singing and listening to praise and worship.

Favorite Young Living product? I use Thieves the most but Sacred Frankincense is very special to me.

Favorite Young Living farm or event? If I had to pick one it would be the Ecuador Farm.

Describe your day using Young Living products:

Morning: Lavender shampoo and Conditioner, Lavender Bath & Shower Gel, Lavender lotion, Thieves AromaBright toothpaste, AromaGuard Mountain Mint Deodorant, Orange Blossom Facial Wash, Satin Facial Scrub Mint, ART toner and Renewal Serum, Sheerlumé, Boswellia Wrinkle Cream, L' Brianté lip gloss, Progessence Plus, EndoFlex, Slique Essence, Stress Away, Peppermint, NingXia Red and Nitro, Balance Complete, Sulfurzyme, BLM, EndoGize, Super B, Digest + Cleanse, Essentialzyme, OmegaGize3, Thieves, Sacred Frankincense, Lime, Orange, Deep Relief, PanAway, Aria Diffuser, Oola Balance

Afternoon: Citrus Fresh, Thieves Household Cleaner, hand sanitizer, spray, foaming hand soap, mints and oil. NingXia Red and Nitro, Essentialzyme, Digest + Cleanse, Balance Complete, Sulfurzyme, BLM, Slique Oil and Bar, Lavender, Purification, Aria Diffuser, Peppermint, Motivation, EndoFlex, Oola Grow, Sacred Frankincense.

Evening: Sulfurzyme, BLM, Essentialzyme, Digest + Cleanse, DiGize, Peppermint, Orange Blossom Facial Wash, ART Refreshing Toner, Renewal Serum, Light Moisturizer and Creme Masque, Progessence Plus, EndoFlex, Lavender, Stress Away, Peace & Calming, Life 5, ImmuPro, Thyromin, Sacred Frankincense, Thieves and R.C.

What does Young Living mean to you? The Lord has used Young Living to bring our family freedom and abundance of health, time, and money, so that we are now WELL able to fulfill His calling on our lives and abundantly bless others. We are now living our dreams and learning to dream BIGGER!

Shannon Hudgens
Diamond, Texas

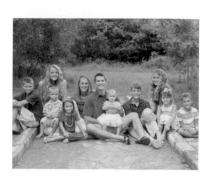

Young Living member since? 2010
Spouse: JD Hudgens
Age: 35
Hobbies: Health and nutrition, reading, every kind of sport, photography, learning
Favorite Young Living product? Frankincense
Favorite Young Living product to gift? Lavender
Favorite Young Living farm or event? The Retreats

Describe your day using Young Living products:

Morning: NingXia Red, Nitro, MindWise, Longevity oil internally and Digest + Cleanse alternated with Life 5, Orange Blossom Facial Wash, ART Renewal Serum, Thieves AromaBright toothpaste, Idaho Blue Spruce (before workout), Peppermint (during/after workout) and after the workout and throughout the day I use Ortho Sport or Ortho Ease massage oil. I like to wear Highest Potential as perfume.

Afternoon: 5-6 drops citrus oil in water with stevia, DiGize with meals, more NingXia, Super C chewables. Diffusing oil of choice, which is always changing, Thieves hand soap and oils all day to fit the need at hand.

Evening: OmegaGize, MultiGreens, Master Formula (alternated with others), Detoxzyme, Sacred Frankincense, Lavender and or Cedarwood on my scalp, Lavender foaming soap, Morning Start shower gel, Lavender shampoo, Orange Blossom face wash, ART masque (once a week), diffuse oil(s) of choice when sleeping—always changing, Progessence Plus and Clary Sage or SclarEssence worn like perfume and on insides of my feet, Thieves toothpaste, Joy or Aroma Life over my heart.

When Traveling: Raindrop before I leave, Longevity oil internally, Inner Defense (or make my own capsule), EndoFlex topically on thyroid points, Melrose around ears (if traveling by plane), Thieves spray and hand sanitizer, Peace & Calming, Stress Away, Frankincense, Melissa, Highest Potential, Harmony.

What does Young Living mean to you? It means freedom and empowerment. It welcomes freedom to walk in the wellness we we're designed to live in, the freedom from financial debt and freedom for the rat-race system. Young Living equips & empowers us with the tools that are needed in life for abundance and wellness in all areas of life.

Shannon Hudson

Diamond, Michigan

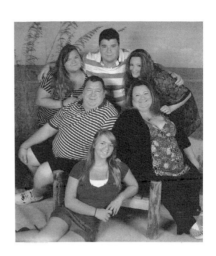

Young Living member since? February 2007
Spouse: Brian Hudson
Age: 46
Favorite Young Living product?
Deep Relief
Favorite Young Living farm or event?
International Grand Convention

Describe your day using Young Living products:

Morning: I keep a basket of oils by my bed and apply them before I even get out of bed: Awaken, Magnify Your Purpose, Believe and EndoFlex. Then I take a scoop each of ICP & JuvaPower. Thieves AromaBright toothpaste, mouthwash and floss. Then Dragon Time shower gel, Lavender shampoo and conditioner and Orange Blossom Facial Wash. ART Refreshing Toner and moisturizer. AromaGuard Mountain Mint Deodorant. Lavender Hand & Body Lotion when I shave. Progessence Plus on midsection and Marjoram, Copaiba, Idaho Balsam Fir, Deep Relief and Wintergreen on arms, legs, neck and shoulders. I also use Lavender Lip Balm throughout the day.

Afternoon: I never stop applying oils. I wear diffuser jewelry. NingXia Red, MindWise, Mineral Essence, Rehemogen, Longevity, EndoGize, OmegaGize, Sulfurzyme, Super B, Super Cal, Essentialzymes 4 and Thyromin are all part of my afternoon. We also take several dietary oils in a shot glass of water with raw honey. I usually take a Nitro in the middle of the afternoon.

Evening: We enjoy NingXia Red as a dessert. I use ART Gentle Cleanser and either ART Masque or Sandalwood Cream. I also apply oils to my feet. Cedarwood inhaled. Dream Catcher, RutaVaLa and Transformation, Life 5 and Thyromin.

What does Young Living mean to you? My friend let me use the Raindrop oils February 2007. I hated them! I didn't like the smell. I didn't like that it was a sales company. I didn't like one of the people in her up line. I thought the company was a huge scam. Even with ALL those issues, my life was changed in 45 minutes. The oils literally gave me hope! I knew I would never be the same and I knew people needed the same opportunity I had been given.

Sonya Swan
Diamond, Iowa

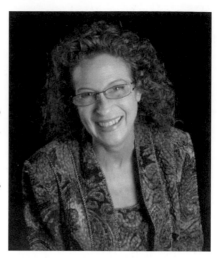

Young Living member since? October 2006

Age: 47

Hobbies: Anything that will empower me to grow and teach others. Teaching about essential oils, healthy eating or matters of faith.

Favorite Young Living product? Thieves

Favorite Young Living farm or event? Diamond Trip in France and Croatia

Describe your day using Young Living products:

Morning: AlkaLime, NingXia Red for all that vital nutrition and antioxidant power. Also, Nitro and MindWise! Brain Power, Clarity, Sulfurzyme and Essentialzyme first thing in the morning to get my digestive system up and running! Any supplement Young Living has I have on my shelf and use as I want to support a particular area.

Afternoon: More NingXia and Nitro and whatever oils I feel like using during the day!

Evening: I use Aroma Life EVERY day and carry it with me all the time. I also use Frankincense, Ocotea, Dill and occasionally Peppermint or DiGize. Detoxzyme to assist with detoxification during the sleeping hours, ImmuPro for overall immune support. These are fairly constant; the rest of oils and supplements may vary from day to day.

When Traveling: Thieves, DiGize, Purification (really the whole everyday oil kit) along with my favorites. NingXia packed in every nook and cranny as well as Nitro. AlkaLime is my other new staple. Life 5 is a must!

What does Young Living mean to you? Freedom. Freedom may be different things for different people.

What is your favorite clean eating meal? Spinach guacamole!

Stacie Hartzler
Diamond, Missouri

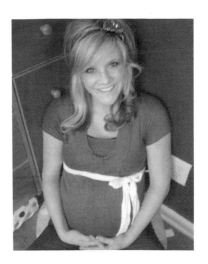

Young Living member since? February 2013
Spouse: Reuben Hartzler
Age: 28
Hobbies: Knitting, cooking, reading, and hiking with family
Favorite Young Living product? AlkaLime
Favorite Young Living farm or event? Grand Convention

Describe your day using Young Living products:

Morning: Wash my face with the ART line plus Beauty Serum mixed with shea butter. Brush my teeth with AromaBright Thieves toothpaste, floss with Thieves dental floss, rinse with Thieves mouthwash. Apply Stress Away on the base of my neck, Peace & Calming on my wrists and Joy over my heart. I also drink a big glass of water with Lemon oil, 2 ounces of NingXia Red, OmegaGize, MultiGreens, a NingXia Nitro, Life 5, Mineral Essence, and a Super C chewable.

Afternoon: Another big glass of water with Lemon and Spearmint, apply Clarity to the sides of my neck, make a smoothie with Balance Complete. Throughout the morning and afternoon I wash my hands with Thieves hand soap and I will have most likely cleaned something with Young Living Thieves cleaner!

Evening. I often took a big glass of water with AlkaLime in it to sip on to help with occasional reflux from being pregnant. I often apply DiGize to my belly to help with my body's digestion. Dinner will most likely have some form of essential oil in it. If it is an evening that I take a shower, I will wash my hair with Copaiba Vanilla shampoo and conditioner! I will also use one of the super awesome bars of soap that Young Living carries! At night, I always diffuse something like Nutmeg, RutaVaLa, Lavender, Cedarwood or Sandalwood!

What does Young Living mean to you? Young Living has changed my life on more than one level. As far as health goes, I have always considered myself pretty healthy because I would never get sick... I didn't realize there was a WHOLE different world of health that I was missing out on! Mentally, physically, emotionally and spiritually, I am so much healthier since choosing Young Living! It has given me an outlet as a stay at home mom to minister to so many other women doing what I LOVE to do!

Stacy McDonald
Diamond, Texas

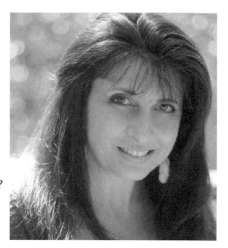

Young Living member since? 2010
Spouse: James McDonald
Age: 48
Hobbies: Writing, cooking, traveling and homeschool mom.
Favorite Young Living product? Vetiver
Favorite Young Living farm or event? Diamond Retreat

Describe your day using Young Living products:

Morning: Progessence Plus, Sulfurzyme, True Source, BLM, Thyromin, Essentialzymes-4, Life 5. Oils of choice for the morning (Vetiver, Present Time, Lady Sclareol, Sandalwood, Common Sense, Frankincense or Abundance), Sensation lotion, ART skin care, Thieves toothpaste and mouthwash, two ounces of NingXia Red.

Afternoon: Two ounces NingXia Red, Essentialzymes-4, Sulfurzyme, oil of choice layered with Sensation lotion (I do this all day long)

Evening: Progessence Plus, Essentialzyme, AlkaLime, ART skin care system, Wrinkle Cream, Wolfberry eye cream, Mineral Essence, Freedom Kit or one of the following: Frankincense, Sara, Vetiver, Lady Sclareol, or Sandalwood, Sensation body lotion.

What is your favorite clean eating meal? I love, love, love salads – good salads! My dream salad has a mix of red and green leafy lettuces, red onion, avocado, beets, cucumber, heirloom tomatoes, asparagus, hearts of palm, garlic scapes, and feta cheese. All topped with a homemade vinaigrette and served alongside a rich cup of creamy, homemade tomato basil soup!

Star Moree

Diamond, Minnesota

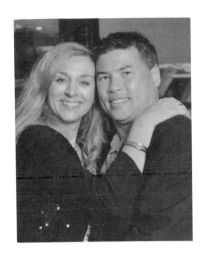

Young Living member since? January 1998

Spouse: David Moree

Age: 47

Hobbies: Our children's activites: figure skating and hockey. Being the "Mom-ager" for our daughter's figure skating, part-time figure skating dress designer, dance Mom

Favorite Young Living product? Stress Away and Thieves

Favorite Young Living product to gift?

Christmas Spirit with diffuser necklace

Favorite Young Living farm or event? St. Maries Lavender Farm

Describe your day using Young Living products:

Morning: Two ounces of NingXia Red and Nitro diluted with water with a 4-6 drops of Mineral Essence to chase down our favorite supplements. These includes Sulfurzymes-4 capsules, MultiGreens, True Source, OmegaGize or MindWise, one Thyromin, Vitamin D3 and ionic and molecular iodine. Stress Away in my lotion! Stress Away and other oils on our feet!

Afternoon: Two ounces of NingXia Red with Nitro, Mineral Essence as above. I also repeat Sulfurzyme and MultiGreens, Life 5 along with adding D3 and ionic and molecular iodine.

Evening: Oil up for relaxation: Peace & Calming and Stress Away.

What does Young Living mean to you? Young Living has been a life changing transformation. I thought I had learned about health in college and graduate school, but I now realize we cannot fool mother nature. I have gone back to my roots and what my Grandma taught me was the right thing for myself and my family! I have met some of the wisest people on the planet in Young Living! I have many mentors in Young Living to look up to, perhaps more than at any other time in my life! I feel that my life has been truly blessed by Young Living and all of our Young Living family! I am grateful for the years leading up to discovering Young Living as the journey of discovery has helped me to be a better person and have more understanding of our world!

Tan Kai Hiang

Diamond, Singapore

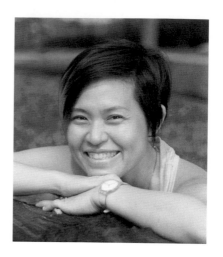

Young Living member since: 2007
Spouse: Sheena Ling
Age: 40
Hobbies: Painting, Hanging with friends
Children: None
Favorite YL product? Peppermint!
Favorite YL product to gift someone?
Lavender or Peppermint.

Describe your day using Young Living products:

Morning: AlkaLime, two ounces of Ningxia Red, Sulfurzyme, BLM, CortiStop. For my laundry I use Thieves Household Cleaner, Baking Soda with Lemon or Peppermint. OolaFaith or Frankincense for worship and quiet time with God. Diffuse any oils that get me going.

Afternoon: 2 ounces of Ningxia Red, Essentialzymes-4 with meal, Essentialzyme between meals. Deep Relief after having worked at computer for a while. Diffuse any oils in car in traveling

Evening: Shower with Lavender Mint shampoo and conditioner. Bath gel base + Transformation oil. ART cleanser or Orange Blossom cleanser (occasionally Satin facial scrub). I use Sandalwood or Frankincense on face with ART moisturizer or ART Renewal Serum and alternate with Sheerlumé. After Shower: Clove, Lavender, Frankincense over chest area. JuvaCleanse over liver, DiGize on stomach, Nutmeg on Adrenals. At bedtime: Cedarwood or Valor. RutaVaLa if I need a good rest. Allerzyme or Detoxzyme. 15 drops of DiGize in a capsule. Thyromin, Progessence Phyto Plus.

What does Young Living mean to you? The heartbeat of Young Living is truth and love. Truth: Gary is always about discovering the truth and making sure others are taught the truth. The journey in using the oils cannot but bring you to a place of seeing the best and the most authentic you. Love: This resonates in all areas that Young Living tries to do; for not just the people who are using the oils but also the entire community around us.

Teresa Gingles

Diamond, Texas

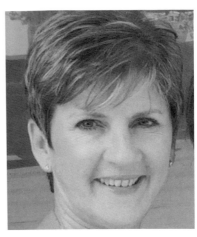

Young Living member since? 2001
Spouse: David Gingles
Age: 59
Hobbies: Bicycling, grandchildren
Favorite Young Living product?
NingXia
Favorite Young Living farm or event?
St. Maries Farm

Describe your day using Young Living products:

Morning: Orange Blossom face wash, Thieves AromaBright toothpaste, floss, mouthwash, Progessence Plus, SclarEssence, ART toner, ART Renewal Serum, Boswellia Wrinkle Cream, Sheerlumé, Lavender lip balm, Lavender Mint shampoo and conditioner, Young Living bath gel, Thieves hand soap, oils on the bottom of our feet. Sulfurzyme, NingXia Red, Essentialzymes-4, Power Meal & Balance Complete (I use one scoop of each in a smoothie), Super C, Longevity, Life 5, Lemon in water.

Afternoon: NingXia Red and Nitro, Essentialzymes-4, Clarity oil, Thieves household cleaner, Thieves toothpaste, Super C, Various oils for any given situation.

Evening: Progessence Plus, Lavender. Same products as the morning regimen. Vetiver, Breathe Again or RC, Dream Catcher, Sulfurzyme, Thyromin, Life 5, OmegaGize.

When Traveling: Thieves hand purifier, Thieves spray and many oils! We spent a month in Europe in April and I had 120 NingXia packets and many other products shipped ahead of us.

What does Young Living mean to you? Young Living meant a new beginning for us in health and finances. I had not had a job since I married in 1975. No one would have hired me for more than a minimum wages but Young Living gave us opportunity few people will ever experience. Health, Wellness and Abundance truly says it all!

What is your favorite clean eating meal? Fresh mustard greens, tomatoes and purple hull peas.

Dr. Thomas Reed

Diamond, Texas

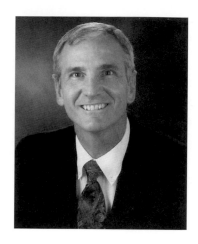

YL member since? 2006

Spouse: Evangeline Reed

Age: 65

Hobbies: Blueberry farming, organic gardening, photography, biking, swimming, weight training, researching health related topics.

Favorite Young Living product? Nitro

Favorite Young Living farm or event? Global Leadership Cruise and Ecuador Farm

Describe your day using Young Living products:

Morning: I am up with the sun and take Nitro, Balance Complete/Power Meal drink three days a week, NingXia Red with Tangerine and Ocotea, OmegaGize, Longevity, Sulfurzyme, shower with Sensation shower gel (yes, I love the smell). Brush teeth with homemade Young Living oil-infused toothpaste, underarm deodorant with Thieves Dentarome Plus Toothpaste or a new oil infused home deodorant stick developed by our fifteen year old son—really nice! Then I put on Shutran, Valor, Sandalwood, Blue Cypress and Cedarwood to go see patients (as a foot and ankle surgeon and specialist).

Afternoon: Refresh with Shutran and whatever else the day calls for.

Evening: Sandalwood, Orange, Frankincense oils in a base of argan oil and hyaluronic acid and ART products.

When Traveling: We take as much of the above as we can in smaller containers of course. We also take as many other oils as we can fit into a one quart plastic bag,

What does Young Living mean to you? Young Living is a way of life for our family. It is a large piece of the puzzle that makes me who I am. It fits very well into the bigger God-centered picture that permeates my life. Young Living is not only a company with great natural health products – for me, it is also a conduit to help bring the message of Jesus Christ into the lives others. The heart of the company is about loving others through sharing. Wellness, Purpose, and Abundance is not just a slogan. It can reveal who we are or who we choose to become, our capacity and desire to grow, and to share God's love with others no matter how small or large.

What is your favorite clean eating meal? Young Living Einkorn pancakes, fresh farm eggs scrambled with raw organic Monterey Jack cheese, diced fresh tomatoes, and fresh organic spinach, chicken and sage sausage. NingXia Red with a splash of Tangerine oil, fresh cantaloupe.

Tina Ciesla
Diamond, Alabama

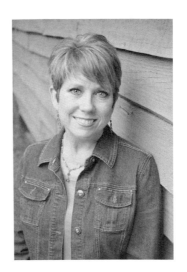

Young Living member since? 2013

Spouse: Paul Ciesla

Age: 47

Hobbies: Homeschool mom, hobby farm (garden, eggs, milk), cheese making, volleyball and cheer mom

Favorite Young Living product? Lavender

Favorite Young Living farm or event? Ecuador

Describe your day using Young Living products:

Morning: ART cleanser, ART toner, Lavender and Frankincense essential oils with a little ART Renewal Serum on face, neck and hands. Then Sheerlumé and Wolfberry Eye Cream. Thieves Dentarome Ultra Toothpaste followed by Thieves mouthwash. I use Lavender Mint shampoo and conditioner (also a great shaving cream). NingXia Red, Nitro and 3 drops of Orange essential oil. Then Master Formula, Super C, and Allerzyme. I use Balance Complete in a smoothie sometimes adding Lemon essential oil. Lavender, Lemon, & Peppermint in a capsule. I love to diffuse either Citrus Fresh, Believe or Joy in my office. In the barn, we use Thieves Household Cleaner as a teat spray on the dairy goats, morning and evening.

Afternoon: NingXia Nitro. Still diffusing in the office. If it is housekeeping day, I am using Purification in my vacuum, Thieves Household Cleaner all over the house. If it is dog washing day, I use Animal Scents shampoo, Purification, and RepelAroma.

Evening: Diffuse Peace & Calming on the nightstand. I apply Valor on the bottom of my big toes and Progessence Plus on the inside of my ankles I repeat my skin care regimen. Thieves toothpaste and mouthwash. I take Life 5 before bed.

What does Young Living mean to you? Young Living has completely changed our lives. The education we have received has deepened our passion for taking care of ourselves. Our family has become closer because Young Living has become a family business. Our children have discovered the love of travel through Young Living. The abundance that overflows from our Young Living business has enabled us to become debt free while allowing us to give to our church and others like never before.

Verick Burchfield

Crown Diamond, Missouri

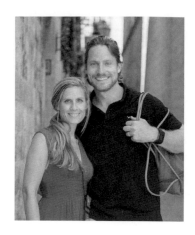

Young Living member since? 2011
Spouse: Crystal Burchfield
Age: 40
Hobbies: Running, outdoors, beekeeping
Favorite Young Living product?
NingXia Red
Favorite Young Living farm or event?
The farm in Provence, France

Describe your day using Young Living products:

Morning: NingXia Red, MindWise, Mineral Essence, Sulfurzyme, Thyromin, Super B, and Shutran

Afternoon: Breathe Again, Motivation

Evening: Cedarwood

When Traveling: Thieves essential oil, Thieves spray and sanitizer. Tons of NingXia Red and Nitro.

What does Young Living mean to you? Young Living means being able to share wonderful products that are healthy for my family and others. When you can impact the health of a family for the better then you have changed a generation. Young Living makes this available to those who use their products. We have been blessed by the leadership, the friendships and the quality, as well as the people involved in this amazing company.

What is your favorite clean eating meal? My favorite meal is fresh vegetables with grilled chicken. Add in some arugula and avocado and it's perfect.

Wendy Mercure

Diamond, Washington

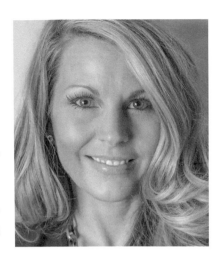

YL member since? June, 2013

Age: 40

Hobbies: My husband is in medical school and I have three little boys. We don't have much time for hobbies at present.

Favorite Young Living product? Frankincense

Favorite Product to Gift? Lavender

Favorite Young Living farm or event? I loved the Silver Retreat last year in Idaho.

Describe your day using Young Living products:

Morning: NingXia Red. Orange Blossom face wash. Frankincense and sometimes other oils neat on the face.

Afternoon: OmegaGize. It's usually time for Stress Away or Joy in the diffuser. At this point one or both of the bigger boys require Lavender oil. My husband Tyson uses En-R-Gee throughout the day to for mental acuity and focus. A little Brain Power under the tongue for good measure.

Evening: Young Living's bath and body products for the kids. Peace & Calming for everyone, too.

When Traveling: Inner Defense! I pack as many oils as I can. And we use lots of Valor.

What does Young Living mean to you? This is incredibly difficult to answer! Young Living means I don't live as a prisoner in my old ways. Young Living means I have a purpose outside of my family; I was meant to help others. Young Living also means security and health. I've never been happier. God put Young Living in our life.

What is your favorite clean eating meal? We eat very simple foods. Organic meat and chicken, veggies and fruit when possible.

Troy Amdahl
Oola Guru, Arizona

What does your day look like using Young Living products?

Morning: OolaGrow every day and OolaFitness for workouts. A shot of NingXia Red. Young Living shampoo.

Afternoon: More OolaGrow and the entire seven oils of the Infused collection based on what "F" of Oola I am working on that day.

Evening: OolaBalance. A shot of NingXia Red.

Dave Braun
Oola Seeker, Utah

What does your day look like using Young Living products?

Morning: NingXia shot every morning. OolaGrow early in the day as well as the Infused kit based on what I'm working on. Right now, I'm using OolaFitness pre- and post-workout.

Afternoon: Blue Spruce oil 2–3 times a day. In the past I've used Copaiba, Lemongrass, Frankincense and Peppermint 3–4 times a day to support my body during times of physical strain and stress.

Evening: I use OolaFaith every evening and diffuse OolaFamily in the dining room and living room. I also use OolaBalance in the evenings.

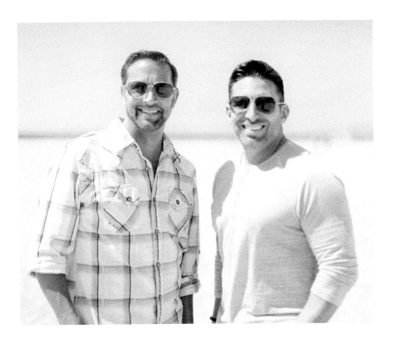

Troy, Oola Guru (left) and Dave, Oola Seeker (right)

What does Young Living mean to the Oola guys?

The mission of Young Living includes Wellness, Purpose and Abundance. The mission of Oola is to change the world with a word by helping people see the purpose inside them and bring out their greatest potential by balancing and growing their lives. This is living their OolaLife.

The lifestyle of Young Living and the lifestyle of Oola are really designed to do the same thing. That is why there is such great synergy between our two companies and why we chose to work with Young Living.

Nikki Davis

Sr. Director of Global Philanthropy
Young Living Corporate

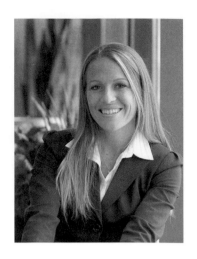

When did you begin with Young Living?
April 2014

Spouse: Awesomeness somewhere out there!

Hobbies: Anything outdoors (hiking, camping, swimming, skiing, running, biking), learning about cultures and history, snorkeling, traveling, connecting with people, being with children

Favorite Young Living product?
Frankincense and NingXia Red

Favorite Young Living farm or event? Ecuador Farm and Foundation Service Trips **Describe your day using Young Living products:**

Morning: Young Living shampoo, conditioner, and body lotion, Thieves toothpaste, Frankincense, Royal Hawaiian Sandalwood and Boswellia Face cream on my face. Thieves, Valor, Stress Away, EndoFlex, JuvaFlex, Grapefruit, Pure Protein Complete smoothie, Grapefruit Lip Balm, NingXia Red, Sulfurzyme, Wolfberry Crisp, Life 5 MindWise. I diffuse different oils all day in the office. Lemon in my water all day, Thieves soap and Hand Sanitizer all day.

Afternoon: Frankincense, Cedarwood, Valor, Stress Away, En-R-Gee, Essentialzymes, MultiGreens, DiGize, Super B, Nitro, Slique Bars, Peppermint, Deep Relief, Gratitude, Believe, Highest Potential.

Evening: Thieves Dish Soap, Laundry Detergent and Cleaner. Copaiba, Helichrysum, RutaVala, Tranquil, Peace & Calming. Thieves Floss and Toothpaste. I use Frankincense, Royal Hawaiian Sandalwood and Boswellia Wrinkle Cream on my face.

What does Young Living mean to you? Wow. Young Living has given me the oppor- tunity to live my purpose and my dream. It allows me to take care of my body and soul in the way that it needs. I never thought it was possible to love my job as much as I do. Young Living provides me the opportunity to associate with people that inspire me to be a better person, with giant hearts and a firm commitment to making the world a better place. Together with our members and corporate staff, it allows me to use my experience and training to empower and bless the lives of others. The people and cul- ture of Young Living feels like home.

Jared Turner

Chief Marketing Officer
Young Living Corporate

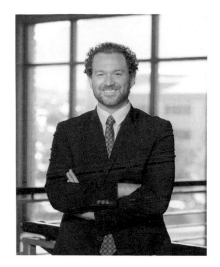

When did you begin with Young Living?
June 2012

Spouse: Felicia Turner

Hobbies: Scuba diving, snowboarding, ornithology

Favorite Young Living product?
Protein Complete, Shutran, Valor

Favorite Young Living product to gift?
Diffuser with Citrus Fresh

Favorite Young Living farm or event? Winter Harvest and Highland Flats

Describe your day using Young Living products:

Morning: Young Living shampoo, Shutran as after shave, Pure Protein Complete shake.

Afternoon: I will use Peppermint and diffuse citrus oils all day long.

Evening: Diffuse Lavender and I rub oils on my son before bed.

When Traveling: Inhale Valor constantly, I use the Bon Voyage Travel Pack.

What does Young Living mean to you?
It is more than a job; it's my life. I and my family's lifestyles are directly affected by Young Living culture and its products. Gary's vision and passion have inspired me from the beginning. We share a love of nature, healthy living and general passion for discovery and life. I've seen countless people's lives changed thanks to Young Living. It's a true movement for good and I'm so happy to be a part of it.

What is your favorite clean eating meal?
Grass-fed beef salad from Cubby's (local Utah restaurant).

Travis Ogden

Chief Operations Officer
Young Living Corporate

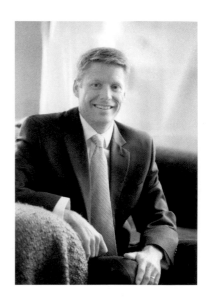

When did you begin with Young Living?
February 2012
Spouse: Holly Ogden
Hobbies: Mountain biking, waterskiing, cycling, snow skiing, off road motorcycling
Favorite Young Living product?
Helichrysum
Favorite Young Living product to gift?
Frankincense

Favorite Young Living farm or event? Ecuador Farm

Describe your day using Young Living products:

Morning: Thieves shampoo, conditioner and soap. Thieves toothpaste & mouthwash. Sulfurzyme and Pure Protein Complete.
Afternoon: Diffuse: Idaho Blue Spruce, Citrus Fresh, Melissa. Apply: Stress Away, Shutran, Valor. Take: Life 5, NingXia Red, Nitro or Zyng every other day.
Evening: Essentialzyme, Prostate Health, Thieves toothpaste & mouthwash.

When Traveling: Bon Voyage Travel Pack, Thieves, Thieves sanitizer, Valor, Peppermint, Lavender, Idaho Blue Spruce, Helichrysum.

What does Young Living mean to you?
Young Living, to me, is more than products, more than even a lifestyle. It is a movement of awareness towards greater health and wellness. Young Living is about helping other people on their pursuit of greater Wellness, Purpose and Abundance. It is a community of people wanting to support each other in this effort.

What is your favorite clean eating meal?
Fish and salad of all kinds with green veggies.

Mary Young

CEO and Co-Founder
Young Living Essential Oils

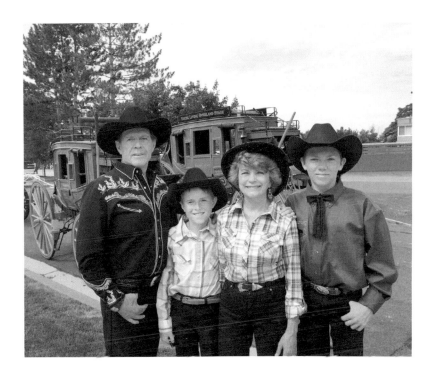

From left: Gary, Josef, Mary and Jacob Young, Founders of Young Living.

What is your favorite Young Living Product?

After living, breathing, sleeping, and eating Young Living for 22 years, I honestly can't say that I have one favorite product. But the products I use the most makes for a long list. Here are a few of them: Essentialzyme, NingXia Red, Nitro, MindWise, Yacon, the new Pure Protein Complete, MegaCal (Gary made this for me when I was pregnant with Josef), Mineral Essence, BLM and MultiGreens.

Describe your day using Young Living products:

I do a shot glass of MindWise every morning with a small dropper full of Frankincense and Helichrysum. I usually do a couple of enzymes (either Essentialzyme or Essentialzymes-4 or sometimes both) with Super B and sometimes Thyromin and EndoGize.

We mix the new Pure Protein in smoothies almost every day: sometimes for breakfast and sometimes in the evening. The boys love the smoothies a lot, and now Josef, the younger one, is becoming our smoothie expert.

I love Yacon and use it whenever I want a little sweetening. With cream cheese frosting, Yacon gives it a little chocolate flavor. We all love it.

You can cover up Mineral Essence by putting it in cold NingXia Red. I also fill an 8-oz. glass with 4 oz. of NingXia and fill the rest with water. I drink it all while I'm working out in the morning.

I also use the ART Cleansing Foam to take off any makeup, and then at night I use different oils. I use singles and blends and they are never the same. It's what suits my fancy. I like the thicker oils on my skin such as patchouli, myrrh, sandalwood, The Gift, Valor, etc. You just have to experiment and see what you like. I am really liking Inner Child on my face and have been using that a lot. Forgiveness also feels wonderful on the skin.

We also love Lavender, Frankincense, Copaiba, RutaVaLa, Light the Fire, DiGize, Melrose, Idaho Balsam Fir, Idaho Blue Spruce, and now the beautiful Northern Lights Black Spruce that is going into more and more blends.

In the morning, I like Sandalwood or Patchouli on my face with one of our moisturizers layered on top. I really like Sheerlumé, and sometimes I just use that. I also use Progessence Plus as a hand and body lotion as well as using it on my face. It's like getting a double benefit.

Gary loves the same supplements that I do. In the morning, he takes about the same; however, at night he takes several Detoxzyme. He really likes that one and between him, the boys, and me, we could go through a bottle in a week. He usually takes Alka-

Lime at night; and when we eat meat, we always take Essentialzymes-4.

Gary has been using Cool Azul for almost two years, and we were thrilled to finally get it into our inventory. Then when he formulated the gel, which was the first to come out, everyone was excited.

Products such as Ortho Ease and Ortho Sport that we have had for a long time are really helpful now that the boys are playing so many sports, and I always carry Helichrysum in my purse.

Gary uses Highest Potential and Shutran every morning, and now the boys are starting to use them as well. Josef was putting so much Shutran on before school that one of the teachers told me that he had to ask Josef not to use so much because it was so strong. We all had a laugh over that one.

We drink a lot of Slique Tea, and Gary often makes a thermos full that he carries with him all day. We all love the Slique Bars and now especially the one with the chocolate, as well as the new Zyng. I have to hide them from the boys because they will eat too many and drink too much on the spot.

I happen to like the Einkorn Nuggets a lot, and Gary started blending them in the smoothies. It works really well and is very tasty.

The Einkorn products are a staple in our house, and we are anxious for new products to be developed. Josef has to have Einkorn pancakes every morning mixed with walnuts and strawberries and covered with blackberry jam that I make from the blackberries that grow in our garden. Einkorn spaghetti is a big hit at home as well, and Gary loves it, which is amazing because he never liked the "other" spaghetti that I made before we had einkorn.

The boys really chew down on our Frankincense gum and think they don't need to brush their teeth, so I have to constantly remind them; and we all love the Thieves AromaBright toothpaste. Actually, we love all the Thieves products, and I have been very impressed with the laundry soap. I think it's fantastic, especially with all the stuff that the boys bring home on their clothes.

I might just add that the new children's diffusers are becoming very popular. Josef just absolutely loves his Dino, which I was not expecting. I thought he was getting too old for that, but I was wrong.

Naturally, everyone has to figure out what products they like by using them, and no two people are alike and choose the same thing. So you just have to experiment and have fun with everything—like one at a time. It's easy to become overwhelmed because there are so many, but I think slower is better when getting to know Young Living.

What is your favorite farm or Young Living event?

My favorite farm event is Farm Day during convention. It is fun to watch how people react to different things. I love seeing the kids just run and have fun. Jacob and Josef always look forward to seeing their Young Living friends, and we only see them here and there as they run from activity to activity.

Gary loves everything about the farms. He loves to see people experiencing the Seed to Seal process at the distillery and walking the fields touching the plants. He always enjoys the jousting and having fun wherever he can be on a horse. Riding is a great joy to him because that is how he grew up; and coming through such a debilitating accident, he appreciates them even more.

Summer harvests or winter harvests come with distinct differences and challenges, and Gary takes it all on like a new adventure every time, and it's even better when he can share that with others. He loves the farms: digging in the dirt, chipping the trees, and watching the oil come up in the separator. The farms are what Gary is all about, and the products that we have in Young Living today are all a result of that great love.

Chapter 4

My Awesome Twin Pregnancy

I remember the day someone said to me "You are such a fun crunchy mom with all your DIY stuff." I smiled and said, "Ohh… well thank you!?" Realistically, I had no idea what she had just said and it wasn't until months later that I actually learned the definition of "crunchy" and "DIY" … (No, I'm not kidding).

For those still novice to these Generation O terms (the OIL generation), "crunchy" apparently means "completely-healthy-all-natural-organic-homemade-back-to-basics" type of person and of course DIY is "do it your-self"… which can range from repurposing an old dresser to making your own face wash and household cleaner.

I was transitioning and transforming my entire life and lifestyle. I became completely dedicated to checking the ingredients on EVERYTHING and learning all I could on the effects of food, oils, chemicals, etc. on our bodies. It was liberating! I lost a lot of extra weight, my hair, nails and skin had never looked better, and I felt amazing overall.

However, even with all these awesome changes in our family, nothing could have prepared me for what happened next…

We were moving our household of eight across the state and I had been busy, busy, busy. I realized something wasn't exactly normal, so I took a pregnancy test to learn that I was unexpectedly pregnant! How exciting!

Everything was perfect; my body was working great… the pregnancy seemed totally normal. I had my first ultrasound and they confirmed the BABY was doing good… with a nice, strong heartbeat. They saw nothing unusual. I went back between ten and eleven weeks for another viability scan and the ultrasound tech put a clear, huge picture up on the screen of what she was seeing. After about two seconds we both at the same time said "WHAT?" … she said, "Umm… did you KNOW?! There are TWO!!!"

#OMGoodness #WHATTT #FreakOutMoment

After the initial shock, tears and calls… we set out to have the best pregnancy ever.

On a side note, as a leader in Young Living, I get phone calls, messages, and emails all the time about what oils and Young Living products are safe, effective and good to use during pregnancy. Let me just say right now that I am a mom. I am a self-taught essential oil enthusiast and loyal Young Living member. My bachelor's degree is not in essential oil study. I am not a doctor, a midwife, or even an aromatherapist. Thus, I cannot treat, prescribe, diagnose, or otherwise advise people on oil usage in that capacity.

However, I will tell you that the more I study, read about and use Young Living essential oils, the more confident I am in their safety and effectiveness for my family. When you give your body what it needs, it works better. Pregnancy is definitely a delicate season of life, but not a medical condition. Also, I referred to Debra Raybern's book *Gentle Babies* for ideas during my twin pregnancy.

I learned that oils work with my body and my baby's bodies and though, yes, moderation is key and it's up to each woman to decide, I personally wasn't worried about having any complications because of using oils or oil-infused products. I ascribe to the French model of aromatherapy, so what I used comes from my studies in that school of thought.

Months 1 & 2:

It was August and September. I was excited but already starting to feel distracted and more tired. I drank a LOT of NingXia and Nitro during these months because we were moving, and most of this time I didn't even know I was pregnant yet! I was also taking Master Formula every day.

Months 3 & 4:

Have you ever heard of hyperemesis gravidarum? If not, go Google it. I had it, and bad. I could hardly get out of bed because every smell made me nauseous. I couldn't keep any food down. I buried my head in my pillow so my husband could rub oils on my feet. I hated every smell, and everything I ever touched or used, or all the people I once loved... haha. Ok maybe not THAT bad, but I *was* miserable. And the only thing I could sometimes stomach was chopped ice with a few drops of Lemon and a little bit of NingXia mixed in. I ate what I could and tried to stay hydrated. I slept a LOT! Some days I smelled Peppermint oil from the bottle and it helped for a few hours. I say this to say that, realty is, even with oils, natural products, a healthy lifestyle, etc. pregnancy is still just pregnancy… and my body was changing—fast!

Months 5 & 6:

This was the most fun season of my pregnancy! I was very big. Measuring around 5-10 weeks ahead already and feeling quite large. I was determined to have a natural VBAC (vaginal birth after cesarean) using oils and a doula at the hospital. I was walking and by this time I was drinking six, eight, even ten ounces of NingXia a day, depending on the day. At the end of month four I started OmegaGize, MultiGreens, Super C Chewable, Master Formula, and Longevity.

I started using oils like Aroma Life, Lemon and Ocotea. I diffused oils all the time, every day. I just used what I felt led to use… and often it was the more mild oils (ones that can be used neat).

I used the Thieves line of products for my home and the only shampoo and conditioner I liked during pregnancy was the Copaiba Vanilla. The ART line kept my face looking good and hydrated, even when my hormones were changing. This is around the time I fell in LOVE with Sheerlumé!

I was eating as much whole food as I could… but I really craved chocolate all the time. So I tried to find chocolate that didn't have high fructose corn syrup and was organic. I love the chocolate bars from the Young Living Christmas catalog!

Months 7 & 8:

I began craving chopped ice. I could eat it five times a day. I would freeze water in ice cube trays with a little NingXia in each cube. Then I'd throw a few ice cubes in the blender for about 20 seconds and scoop it into a cup and eat with a spoon. YUMMY. (Looking back it doesn't sound good at all, but at the time I would wake up in the night craving it. I know that meant I was probably low in iron, but I *was* building two humans).

I used a lot of Stress Away roll on, Aroma Life on my chest, Lavender lotion with Frankincense, Lavender, Myrrh, Elemi, and Geranium on my belly for my skin.

I loved diffusing citrus oils. I used White Angelica, Peace & Calming, Valor, Motivation, En-R-Gee, and Grounding to stay mentally sane (haha, no seriously, have you ever been pregnant with twins? You feel like your bladder and lungs are punching bags all day long. So you always have to run to the bathroom but then you can't breathe after running because you have no lung capacity left.) It's a beautiful season, but I still needed some "keep me sane" oils.

Month 9:

This month people looked at me as if I had two heads. Really. (And not just on the INSIDE of my belly). I was SO big. Everyone asked "SURELY, PLEASE tell me you are having TWINS?!?" I looked like a beached whale, or as my two year old said, "I think you ate a big, huge balloon." (Thank you, thank you very much).

This month I used Young Living Lavender lotion with Marjoram, Peace & Calming and Stress Away all over my legs to help them relax as I was sleeping.

I drank Lemon in my water a lot to maintain healthy circulation. I also took a capsule of various dietary oils every other day or so.

My doctor was amazed. At my biggest measurement, I measured 55.5 weeks pregnant. I had no swelling, no major complications, and had the two of the most active baby boys the nurses had ever seen on ultrasound!

Labor & Delivery:

I was getting bigger, and bigger and bigger. My doctor was getting a little concerned that the babies were so large. On the last ultrasound they measured their approximate weight at about 7.5 pounds each. The OBGYN I had chosen has been delivering babies since the 1950's. He's very experienced and I trusted his professional opinion. On the day I was 38 weeks and 3 days, I had not dilated or effaced beyond two centimeters and 50% in two weeks. Because of a lot of factors including that this was my attempted VBAC after attempting a natural birth the first time around, we made the tough decision to proceed the following day with a scheduled C-section. I hated to go the surgical route, but I knew it was the right choice for us at the time.

The babies were born in perfect health on May 8, 2015 at 9:19 in the morning. They scored a 9 & 9 and 10 & 10 on the APGAR score. They were an average of seven pounds each (7.3 and 6.13). They were fat, pink, healthy and happy!

They nursed within an hour and I applied Sacred Frankincense to their feet within a few hours after they were born, and then Trauma Life a few hours after that. I continued my NingXia Red and went through an entire bottle within the first three days after their birth. I used ClaraDerm spray on my incision site along with Myrrh and Lavender.

I also used Myrrh and Lavender on the boys' circumcision wound and umbilical cord.

Their first bath at home was with KidScents shampoo and lavender in the water. I used Chamomile oils, Gentle Baby, Lavender, Helichrysum, Frankincense, Myrrh and KidsScents oils on the babies during those first few weeks.

When I went back to get my staples removed from my incision, the nurse actually yelled out "OH MY WORD. THAT LOOKS AMAZING!"

I had a good and easy recovery. It was a real blessing to have Young Living products to prepare my body for delivery as well as encourage a healthy environment in all my systems for post-delivery wellness. It was awesome. I felt empowered. I felt healthy. I felt accomplished to have brought such mighty little baby boys into the world.

Since nursing the twins, I have used all my oils, Young Living products, NingXia Red, Nitro, and supplements faithfully. I am totally in LOVE with Sheerlumé—as it's been my saving grace for my skin during the many long nights that run into the long days. The only oil I avoid in high amounts is Peppermint, which slightly reduces some mom's milk supply and I don't want to risk that with my "little litter" as I affectionately call the twins sometimes while they're nursing. I feel so confident in feeding my babies knowing that I am doing all I can to set them up for a lifetime of health.

A Forever Changed Family

Our family has been forever changed by Young Living. Everything from pregnancies, daily routines around the home, the way we travel, the